Ralf Johannes Radlanski
Contributions to the Development
of Human Deciduous Tooth Primordia

Contributions to the Development of Human Deciduous Tooth Primordia

Prof. Dr. Ralf Johannes Radlanski
Berlin, Germany

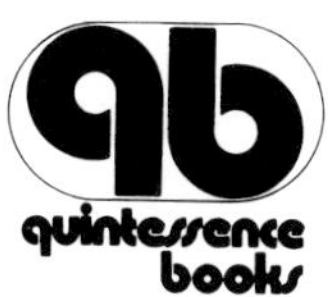

Quintessence Publishing Co, Inc
Chicago, Berlin, London, Tokyo, Moscow, Prague, Sofia, Warsaw

This work was conducted at the Department of Orthodontics (Head: Prof. Dr. Kubein-Meesenburg) of the Dental Institute of the Faculty of Medicine of the University of Göttingen, Germany.

Inaugural dissertation to obtain the "venia legendi", submitted to the Medical Faculty of the Georg August University of Göttingen. Original title: Beiträge zur Gestaltentwicklung menschlicher Zahnanlagen der ersten Dentition.

Publikation of English text supported by the German Research Association.

Author's address:

Prof. Dr. R. J. Radlanski
Freie Universität Berlin
Institut für Klinisch-Theoretische Zahn-, Mund- und Kieferheilkunde
Abt. Mikromorphologie
Aßmannshauser Straße 4–6
D-14197 Berlin (Dahlem)
Germany

Library of Congress Cataloging-in-Publication Data

Radlanski, Ralf Johannes.
Contributions to the development of human deciduous tooth
primordia / Ralf Johannes Radlanski.
p. cm.
Includes bibliographical references.
ISBN 0-86715-261-3
1. Teeth—Embryology. 2. Teeth—Differentation. I. Title
[DNLM: 1. Tooth, Deciduous—embryology.
2. Tooth, Deciduous—growth & development. WU 480 R129b 1993a]
QM311.R3413 1993
611'.013—dc20
DNLM/DLC
for Library of Congress 92-48439
CIP

Lithography: Sixty-Six Lithographic Pte. Ltd., Singapore
Composition, Printing and Binding: Buchdruckerei Loibl, Neuburg

Printed in West Germany

Contents

Preface 9

1 Introduction **11**

1.1 The question 11

1.2 Variety of approaches 12
1.2.1 Evolutionary concepts 12
1.2.2 Genetic approach 13
1.2.3 Embryological experimental research 13
1.2.4 Mechanical interdependencies as cofactors of morphogenesis 13

1.3 Formal development of tooth primordia 13

1.4 Purpose of this study 14

2 Materials, methods, and techniques **17**

2.1 Specimens 17

2.2 Technique of reconstruction 17
2.2.1 Tracing of contours 17
2.2.2 Computer-aided graphic reconstruction 19
2.2.3 Graphic reconstruction compared to construction of solid models 20

3 Findings **21**

3.1 Stage of the dental lamina 21
3.1.1 Maxillary region 21
3.1.2 Mandibular region 23

3.2 Bud stage 24
3.2.1 Early bud stage 24
3.2.1.1 Maxillary region 24
3.2.1.2 Mandibular region 24
3.2.2 Late bud stage 25

3.3 Bud and early cap stage 26
3.3.1 Primordium of i^1 27
3.3.2 Primordium of i^2 27
3.3.3 Primordium of c^1 27
3.3.4 Primordium of m^1 27
3.3.5 Primordium of m^2 28
3.3.6 Primordium of i_1 28
3.3.7 Primordium of i_2 30
3.3.8 Primordium of c_1 30
3.3.9 Primordium of m_1 33
3.3.10 Primordium of m_2 34

3.4 Cap stage 34
3.4.1 Primordium of i^1 37
3.4.2 Primordium of i^2 39
3.4.3 Primordium of c^1 39
3.4.4 Primordium of m^1 39
3.4.5 Primordium of m^2 39
3.4.6 Primordium of i_1 40
3.4.7 Primordium of i_2 40
3.4.8 Primordium of c_1 42
3.4.9 Primordium of m_1 45
3.4.10 Primordium of m_2 45

3.5 Early bell stage 45
3.5.1 Primordium of i^1 46
3.5.2 Primordium of i^2 46
3.5.3 Primordium of c^1 47
3.5.4 Primordium of m^1 48
3.5.5 Primordium of m^2 49
3.5.6 Primordium of i_1 51
3.5.7 Primordium of i_2 51
3.5.8 Primordium of c_1 52
3.5.9 Primordium of m_1 54
3.5.10 Primordium of m_2 56

4 Discussion 63

4.1 Thickening and invagination of the oral epithelium 63

4.2 Laminar stage 63
4.2.1 Pattern of invagination of vestibular and dental laminae 63
4.2.2 *Nebenleiste* and prelacteal lamina 64
4.2.3 Outline of the dental lamina 65

4.3 Bud stage 65

4.4 Cap stage 67

4.5	Bell stage	69
4.5.1	Comparative anatomy of the primordia in the bell stage	69
4.5.2	Assumptions concerning cusp formation	70
4.5.3	Topography of tooth bells and surrounding bone	73
5	**Final remarks**	**75**
5.1	Form of the primordia	75
5.1.1	Early characteristic differences	75
5.1.2	Longitudinal comparison	75
5.2	Topography of dental primordia and their surrounding bone	76
5.3	Morphogenesis of the dental primordia	76
5.4	Methodological compromise	77
6	**Summary**	**79**
7	**References**	**83**
8	**Index**	**87**

Preface

Tooth development as a multifactorial process requires various approaches from different technical directions.
In present times the focus is concentrated on the cellular and biochemical level of differentiation, whereas the question of form has been more neglected. Understanding embryology requires a perception of differentiation of tissue, but of equal importance is recording the changes in the growing form. The classic wax plate reconstruction after histological serial sections could deliver three-dimensional knowledge of the *gestalt* almost a century ago. So the formal development of the tooth primordium over its typical stages, such as lamina, bud, cap, and bell, is well known. It was, however, too time consuming to be pursued much further, with the exception of the great work of Ooe. So in particular our knowledge concerning the development of position and form of the tooth primordia *in relation to their neighboring* hard tissue structures remained rather sparse.
There are several hints that differentiation and development do not act alone within single structures, and there is reason to assume a mutual influence of adjacent structures while both are engaged in the developmental process. So it is necessary to follow the changes of their mutual spatial relationship as well as the changes in each form. This is not only meant to trace evidence of a direct mechanical interaction, but to map the distances that have to be covered between different tissues on the cellular and subcellular level as well.
Today, the omnipresent personal computers and adequate software make it possible to speed up the old method of three-dimensional reconstructions from histological serial sections. So in the present study I am able to present computer-aided graphic reconstructions that show complete dental arches of human embryos and different developmental stages of fetal tooth primordia in relation to adjacent bony structures of maxilla, mandible, and Meckel's cartilage.
Thus it is possible to identify on the micromorphological level the regions where the biochemical processes of tissue differentiation take place. In addition, I understand my study as a further step in shedding light on the interdependency of position and form as a morphogenetic principle.
I hope this book is interesting for research colleagues engaged in the study of dental and oral morphogenesis, and that the illustrations of the dental primordia may be helpful teaching aids for gaining a conception of the interesting developmental processes taking place in every individual.

Ralf J. Radlanski, Berlin

1 Introduction

1.1 The question

"Now these teeth[1] are developed before the flat teeth,[2] in the first place because their function is earlier (for dividing comes before crushing, and the flat teeth are for crushing, the others for dividing), in the second place because the smaller is naturally developed quicker than the larger, even if both start together, and these teeth are smaller in size than the grinders, because the bone of the jaw is flat in that part but narrow towards the mouth. From the greater part, therefore, must flow more nutriment to form the teeth, and from the narrower part less."

–Aristotle, Generation of Animals. Book V 8, quot. acc. to Barnes (1981)

Spatial conditions of tooth development and aspects of onset and duration of development are important issues for Aristotle in this section of his work from *Generation of Animals*. As this quotation shows, the interest in morphogenesis of human teeth is very old, yet it is still an unsolved problem. Despite more than 2,000 years of research,[3] the spatial conditions under which tooth primordia develop and the possible influence exercised by their surrounding structures are still not fully understood and are a primary focus in this study. For Aristotle, the purpose of an organ is one of the main reasons why it is developed by nature. Next to the ontogenetic and phylogenetic way of looking at developmental processes, purpose *(Zweckmäßigkeit)* was considered by Peter (1920) to be one of the causal reasons for morphogenesis. Although teleogic thinking is today very common in explanatory schemes, it must be well emphasized, that *purpose* is attributed to certain organs only by man. There is no convincing mechanism that could explain how morphogenetic processes leading to the formation of a certain organ should be directly influenced by the later purpose of it: a favorable purpose can be recognized only *after* formation of the organ, during its period of usage. It must be clearly stated that there is no link between the philosophic category to which the study of purpose belongs and the physiologic category to which research on morphogenetic processes belongs (Meyer 1926). In evolutionary biology the claim has been described very extensively that natural selection is the main factor that decides whether a certain organ is expressed during morphogenesis or not, since only those organs contribute to survival that serve a favorable purpose. Those that do not are sentenced to perish by selection. A more extensive discussion of this field of questions can be found in Shaw (1924), Brace (1963), Mayr (1963), Ho and Saunders (1971), Starck (1980), Wuketits (1980), and Altner (1981). The embryologist, however, must point out that an organ or a structure that is subjected to natural selection must have been developed *prior to that selection* by morphogenetic processes. Thus, any material that undergoes selection with positive or negative results must have its source of success or failure in morphogenesis.

We all know that the teeth of the human dental arch do look different; we observe the typical incisor, canine, and molar shapes. The expert can be even more precise and is able to distinguish for example different molars and can clearly identify the position of each single tooth within the dental arch.

1. The incisors.
2. The molars. In this study I, however, use the term *flat teeth* for the incisors because they and their primordia (in certain stages) are flat in mesiodistal direction.
3. A comprehensive survey of dental research concerning morphology and morphogenesis is given by Norberg (1929) and, more detailed, by Würtz (1985).

Teeth are a very common example for so-called and putative preadaptional (deBeer 1951) processes of morphogenesis because they develop completely encased by bony structures before they erupt into the oral cavity and in most cases fit together perfectly, serving well-adapted, functional patterns of mastication. It is obvious that the necessities of gnathologic function can neither influence the formation of incisal edges or cusps, nor influence the folding pattern of the inner enamel epithelium or the depository rates of enamel matrix: all of this happens during the embryonic and fetal period of life long before the individual begins to chew.

We may rightly ask, therefore, whether the explanation for adult tooth function could be the other way around: if teeth are not formed in order to fulfill later functional requirements, *function is a consequence of morphogenetic processes*.

The questions that led to this study are: Do the epithelial tooth primordia show specific characteristics of form like the completed teeth do? Are primordia of incisors typically as flat as the completed incisors? If so, what makes them flat? Why are molars relatively larger than other teeth? Is it a question of available space and of the possibility of expansion? Why do molars develop cusps, which enable occlusal interdigitation of cusp and fossa? Is it a question of a folding pattern that is more or less identical in maxillary and mandibular primordia?

It may be speculated that there are mechanical influences like pressure and traction during the process of morphogenesis that contribute to the multifactorial process leading to tooth form.

Because differences of form, of *gestalt*[4] of the tooth primordia, are likely to be expected, this study was designed first to trace the changes of gestalt during the early stages of development, so enabling comparisons of the primordia within the same dental arch. In addition, special attention was paid to the structures that surround the tooth primordia.

4. Unfortunately there is no specific English translation of the German word *gestalt*, which means more than *form, figure, outline*, or *shape*. In the context of this study the term *gestalt* includes the three-dimensional outer appearance of the embryologic formations. Whenever possible, the term *gestalt* is replaced by specific English vocabulary, but in some cases I found it necessary to use *gestalt* with the meaning just described.

Computer-aided three-dimensional reconstructions of serial sections were employed and are reproduced in this book.

1.2 Variety of approaches

1.2.1 Evolutionary concepts

A variety of different approaches have been made to investigate dental development. The most prominent theories about tooth and cusp formation came from evolutionary biology (see Schumacher et al. 1990 for a literature survey), probably because dental enamel is one of the hardest substances of the body and can withstand decay over extensive paleontologic time spans. The evolutionary aspect is elucidated by a sometimes contradictory variety of results and theories. Only the most popular examples of the theory of differentiation (Cope 1883, 1889; Osborn 1892, 1897, 1907; Gregory 1934) and the theory of concrescence (Kükenthal 1892, Röse 1892b, Schwalbe 1894) will be mentioned here. However, besides the fact that these theories are contradictory, evolutionary theories, in general, miss the point of this study: although the existence of a dental evolution should not be denied, it must be stated that this kind of research is a historical discipline. And from this historical, phylogenetic reconstruction (should it be possible at all), we are not able to deduce the ontogenetic mechanisms leading to creation of organic form (Meyer 1926, deBeer 1951, Goll 1972, Blechschmidt 1976). As indicated above, evolution, natural selection, and adaption to altered surroundings, can only be possible if the offspring, which is subjected to selection, is more or less different from its parents. These differences are due to deviating processes, and it is *there* that one must search. The aim of Cope (1871) has not lost relevance during the last century of research: *"Darwin assumes a 'tendency to variation' in nature, and it is plainly necessary to do this, in order that materials for the exercise of a selection should exist. Darwin and Wallace's law is, then, only restrictive, directive, conservative, or destructive of something already created. I propose then to seek for the originative laws by which these subjects are furnished – in other words, for the causes of the origin of the fittest."* (Cope 1871, p 230)

1.2.2 Genetic approach

From the similarities and variations of tooth form, a variety of genetic regularities were derived (Korkhaus 1940, Dahlberg 1945, 1965, Garn et al 1963, Osborne 1967, Fitzgerald 1969, Müller 1975, Garn 1977, Harzer 1987, Schulze 1987), and certain ancestral relationships were concluded from phenotypic data. Therefore these studies are usually understood to enrich the phylogenetic approach. However, it is necessary to distinguish between this kind of "genetics," which is rather another kind of description of morphological patterns, and those contributions to molecular genetics which could bridge the gap between molecular genetics (level of genotype) and, for-example, the folding pattern in space of the epithelium of a tooth primordium (level of phenotype). Although today much work is done in this field of research, the question remains: What kind of variations of the genetic code lead to different metabolic patterns that affect mechanical properties of the developing structures? Properties like stiffness of epithelial layers, mutual adhesion of cell membranes, different elasticity of cellular matrix, may well influence, for example, the folding patterns of the inner enamel epithelium of a tooth bell stage enamel organ.

1.2.3 Embryological experimental research

The border between embryological experimental research and molecular genetics is wide open today, and perhaps important modes of operation and interdependencies leading to formation of the teeth may be found this way. Extensive histochemical studies (for references see Sternberger 1979, Hay 1981, and Diekwisch 1987), as well as recombination and transplantation experiments of epithelial and mesenchymal parts of primordia, have been undertaken (for references see Gaunt and Miles 1967, Kollar and Baird 1969, Thesslef and Hurmerinta 1981). There is one critical remark, however, that must be made concerning the validity of these experiments: if mechanical factors are considered to be of importance during morphogenetic processes, it must be taken into account that these very mechanical interdependencies may be destroyed by experiments that include transplants, injections, or incisions.

1.2.4 Mechanical interdepencies as cofactors of morphogenesis

Today the most commonly held opinion is that there is a DNA sequence programming the development of every single detail of a structure. It must be taken into account that, as epigenetic influences, neighboring structures themselves may be a cofactor of morphogenesis. While growing and expanding, adjacent structures may exercise mutual influence on each other. Grüneberg (1937) showed that in *gray lethal* mice dental development was severely affected because of a defect of bone resorption. This kind of mutual influence that developing structures exercise on each other is, of course, not solely of mechanical nature. We know about the epigenetic influence of chemicals as well, but I only want to point out that pressure and traction as mechanical factors should be taken into consideration, and perhaps they stimulate or inhibit differentiation on a chemical basis. Perhaps Spemann's inductor (1936) can be looked at in this way. Blechschmidt (1948, 1964, 1976, 1978) has drawn attention to an abundance of findings that lead to the conclusion that genetic action can be interpreted as more of a reactive process in morphogenesis than an active process. According to Blechschmidt (1948), the genetic code is used as the reservoir of information that reacts to different situations that constantly arise and change during growth and mutual exercise of stress. This approach, although old (His 1874), demands much more detailed knowledge of the gestalt and spatial arrangement of the different structures forming during morphogenesis.

1.3 Formal development of tooth primordia

The formal development of the tooth primordia covering the stages of the lamina, bud, cap, and bell is sufficiently described (Röse 1891, Leche 1892, Ahrens 1913a, Nilson 1928, Norberg 1929, Meyer 1951, Ooe 1956, 1958, 1959, 1962, 1965, 1971, 1981, Garn and Burdi 1971; surveys by Eidmann 1923, Gaunt and Miles 1967, Thesslef and Hurmerinta 1981, Schroeder 1987, Schumacher et al 1990). The oral epithelium invaginates into the underlying mesenchyme, thus forming a maxillary and a mandibular epithelial lamina. In the anterior region, from this common lamina there arise two laminae, one to form the dental lamina from which the tooth buds arise, the other to form the oral vestibule. In the lateral regions the vestibular lamina is a separate invagination of the oral epithelium. The dental lamina forms 10 swellings, which are called the *tooth buds*. In most cases they bear a central protrusion called the enamel knot (*Schmelzknoten*,[5] Ahrens 1913a). During growth these buds change their appearance into caplike formations. As soon as the margins of the tooth caps bulge and grow further into the depth of the mesenchyme, the stage of the early tooth bell is reached. At this stage the dental epithelium is distinguished as the inner enamel epithelium at the inside of the bell and the outer enamel epithelium at the outside of the tooth bell. In the inner enamel epithelium the cells will later differentiate into ameloblasts, which will secrete matrix proteins as a precursor of the enamel. The mesenchyme underlying the inner enamel epithelium is condensed and will give rise to the formation of dentin and tooth pulp. The outer surface and shape of the tooth crown is created by the deposition of enamel matrix, which is dependent from the developmental movements (ie, movement of the structure or parts of it caused by change of its size and gestalt during development) of the inner enamel epithelium.

The epithelial ridge between the tooth primordia is called the *general dental lamina*. Between the tooth primordium and the general dental lamina there runs another epithelial lamina that Bolk (1913) called the *laterale Schmelzleiste* (lateral enamel lamina). In this way there is formed a mesial and a distal recess, which is bordered by the lateral enamel lamina, the dental lamina, and the primordium itself. The deeper recess is called the enamel niche (*Schmelznische,* Bolk 1913) the more troughlike recess is called enamel trough (*Schmelzmulde,* Meyer 1951). The lateral enamel lamina is a temporary formation that will be reduced toward the late bell stage. Another temporary formation is the *Nebenleiste*[6] of Bolk (1913), which runs parallel to the vestibular lamina in the sulcus between the primordium and the vestibular lamina.

5. Denominations like *Schmelzknoten* - enamel knot (Ahrens 1913a), *Schmelzstrang* - enamel chord (Ahrens 1913a), *laterale Schmelzleiste* - lateral enamel lamina (Bolk 1913), *Schmelznische* - enamel niche (Bolk 1913), and *Schmelzmulde* - enamel trough (Meyer 1951), do not describe precursor structures of the later formed *enamel*, but refer only to the epithelial structures of the early primordium. This nomenclature obviously is not correct, but it is historical and generally accepted.

6. Neben means: next to, and leiste means: lamina.

1.4 Purpose of this study

The question of space during morphogenesis has been considered as early as the 4th century BC by Aristotle, and laboratory research dealing with morphogenesis of tooth primordia has been carried out for more than a century. Nevertheless, it is astounding that today there is insufficient knowledge either to describe the three-dimensional form, or the *gestalt* of the different primordia or to follow the *topogenesis* (developmental movements) in relation to the surrounding structures.

As mentioned, we would expect differences in the gestalt of the early primordia that are in accordance with the gestalt of the completed teeth, and that, in a typical way, are different from another. However, we have lacked sufficient three-dimensional preparations that would allow a comparison of the primordia within the same dental arch and during different developmental stages.

In addition, there are only a few preparations that show the development of the tooth germs with their surrounding structures included. For embryological research, and especially for the question of whether spatial impediment may be a cofactor of morphogenesis, the exact knowledge of the form and its change of gestalt, as well as of position in the topographic arrangement during further development, is an important prerequisite.

It is to address these morphological questions concerning the primordia of the primary dentition of human material that the present study was designed.

Although there are different ways of gaining preparations of tooth primordia, in the present study the classical three-dimensional reconstruction after serial histologic sectioning was chosen.

Because the questions of this study focus on the gestalt, only three-dimensional representations can be of sufficient validity. The interpretation of two-dimensional, single histologic sections may lead to enormous errors because of projection phenomena that are dependent on the plane of section.

Although greatly neglected, the classical construction of solid models from serial sections (Born 1883) has retained its value and justification until today. However, the rapid development of today's personal computers has enabled us to gain graphic reconstructions that can be interpreted in a way similar to interpreting solid reconstructions. Therefore, computer-aided graphic three-dimensional reconstructions, which are easier and less time-consuming to produce, were employed for the present study.

2 Materials, methods, and techniques

2.1 Specimens

Human embryos and fetuses were used for the present study. All material was provided by the collection of the Department of Embryology of the Institute of Anatomy of the University of Göttingen, Germany. The specimens were prepared as serial histologic sections. Only specimens that did not show external indications of malformations were used. Prior to histologic processing, the heads of all specimens were documented by means of stereoscopic photography from the frontal and lateral view. This served as an aid for the alignment of the single sections to form the reconstructions. The size of the embryos and fetuses was measured as crown-rump length (CRL).

The specimens were fixed in Bouin's solution and were transferred into alcohol prior to histologic processing. Depending on size and gross preparation, the specimens were decalcified using the rapid decalcifier RDO (Eurobio S. A., Paris) for 2 to 30 days. Parafin embedding was carried out according to standard histologic procedures: dehydration through increasing concentrations of ethyl alcohol, methyl benzoate, benzyl alcohol, benzol-Paraplast and Paraplast (Paraplast No. 9685–501006, Monoject Scientific Inc, Athy, Ireland). All specimens were cut as 10-μm-thick serial sections, which were then stained by hematoxylin and eosin.

Table 1 List of serial sections

Size of specimen (CRL, in mm)	Catalog number	Plane of section
17	TON 29. 7. 87	sagittal
18	GUS 11. 7. 85	sagittal
21	ALI 7. 7. 85	horizontal
29	OLL 8. 7. 85	sagittal
33	UTE 8. 6. 87	frontal
34	DON 2. 7. 85	frontal
37	DOR 20. 7. 85	sagittal
38	HEI 9. 7. 85	sagittal
40	PAU 5. 7. 87	sagittal
40	ILO 5. 7. 85	sagittal
40	STE 13. 6. 87	horizontal
40	QUI 18. 6. 87	frontal
45	ERN 3. 7. 85	frontal
47	NIN 26. 6. 85	sagittal
53	JOH 30. 6. 85	horizontal
56	LIL 4. 7. 85	horizontal
60	KAL 6. 7. 85	horizontal
64	VER 16. 10. 87	sagittal

2.2 Technique of reconstruction

2.2.1 Tracing of contours

In each section the contours of epithelium, bone, cartilage, vessels, and nerves were determined histologically under the light microscope. The microscope was equipped with a drawing tube that allowed enlargement (X 30 to 130) and tracing of the contours of each section on transparent paper (Gaunt and Gaunt 1978). The drawings were

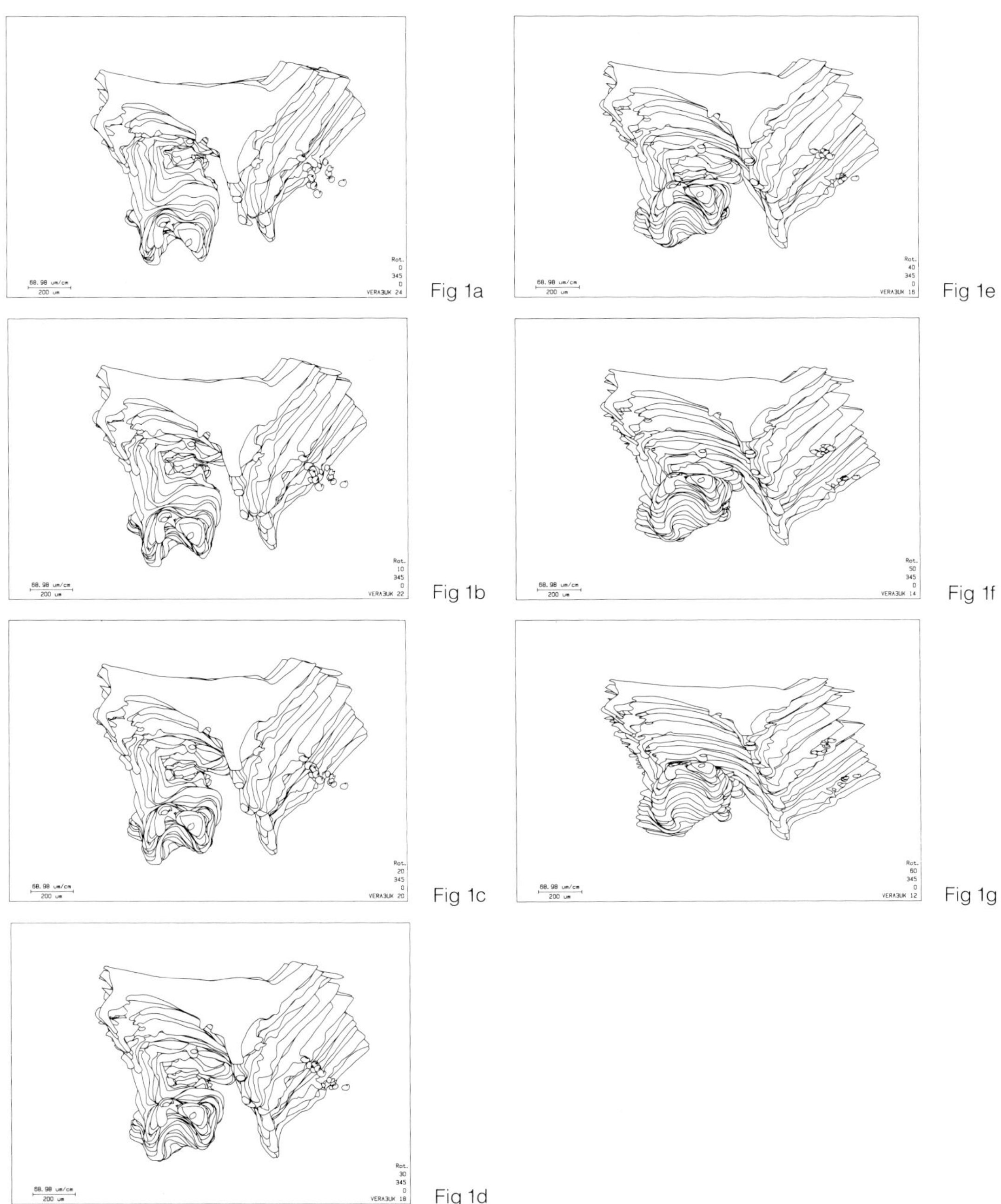

Figs 1 a to g Example of a graphic reconstruction produced as a contour-line plot with the aid of the software HISTOL. Depicted is the right primordium of c_1 of a fetus (64 mm CRL) seen from a lateral aspect (Fig 1 a). In each of the following plots (Figs 1 b to g) the reconstruction is rotated an additional 10° around the x-axis (which lies horizontally and approximately in the center of the reconstruction).

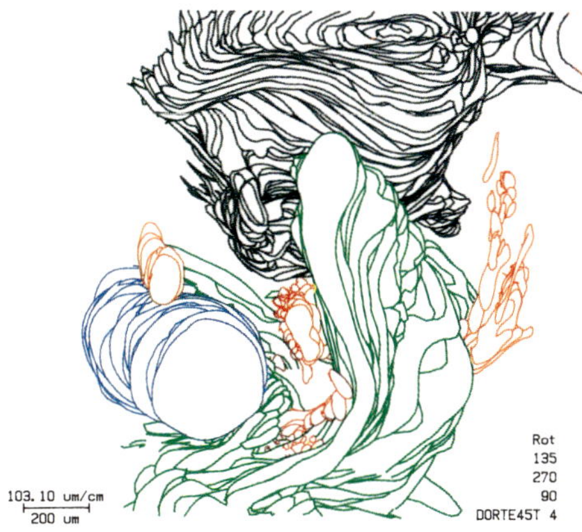

Fig 2 Example of a graphic survey reconstruction produced as a contour-line plot with the aid of the software HISTOL. This plot shows the perioral structures of the right side of a fetus, 37 mm CRL, from a dorsal aspect. The various structures are plotted with different colors (epithelium, black; mandible, green; Meckel's cartilage, blue; nerves, orange; vessels, red) and they are connected as clusters so that they partially hide each other. The software allows one to partially omit various structures.

piled on a light box, and the correct alignment of the single sections was checked using the outer contours of the face, which had been photographed prior to sectioning. In addition, correct alignment of the sections was checked from the reconstructed form of the eyes or Meckel's cartilage.

Automatic scanning of the histologic sections for the present purposes is not yet possible today. A differential diagnosis of the various structures of the histologic material is necessary and cannot be described merely by parameters such as brightness, cell density, or typical contour patterns.

2.2.2 Computer-aided graphic reconstruction

For reconstructions of relatively lesser complexity, the technique of pure graphic reconstruction can be employed (Odhner 1911, Gaunt and Gaunt 1978). Here the contours are drawn in such a way that when all sections are superimposed, the hidden lines are omitted. The result is a representation of the surface as a contour-line plot. If different and distorted coordinate systems are used, it is possible to obtain views that vary slightly from the plane of section. Today it is possible to use computers (Poelmann and Verbont 1985) and personal computers (Gras and Killmann 1983, Gras 1984) for graphic reconstruction, which accelerates the process.

Tooth primordia and their surrounding structures are not too complex to prohibit graphic reconstruction (Radlanski and Jäger 1992) and so for the present study it was possible to use computer-aided graphic reconstruction. In this way it was possible to prepare a greater number of reconstructions, which permitted a comparison of different primordia during several stages.

For the computer-aided three-dimensional reconstruction, the software HISTOL© (H. König, Tübingen, Germany) was employed. The contours of the structures, which had been traced on transparent paper, were entered into an IBM-compatible personal computer via a KONTRON graphic tablet (Digicad). Hardcopies were obtained by means of a six-color plotter (KPL 710, Taxan).

The software HISTOL allows reconstruction of the three-dimensional form and reproduction of it in the "hidden-line-mode" as contour-line maps, as they are known in manual graphic reconstruction techniques. The reconstruction can be rotated on the screen and viewed from almost any direction (Figs 1a to 1g), except 0° rotation to the section plane. In addition to the hidden-line presentation, stereoscopic pairs of plots can be obtained, which were used several times in this study for diagnostic reasons. (The validity of the graphic reconstructions was verified by stereoscopic plots and by several representative solid reconstruction models as well; it was judged that graphic reconstruction, checked by stereoscopic plots, was sufficient for the purpose of this study.) Different structures –

for this study epithelium, maxillary and mandibular bone, cartilage, nerves, blood vessels – can be labelled separately and can be plotted with different colors (Fig 2). In addition, different structures can be temporarily omitted and quickly restored, in order to view structures that are hidden by structures lying closer to the viewer. Further, variable magnifications of details can be obtained.

Because the contour-line plots are not easily interpretable by everyone at first glance, I graphically reworked the plots according to Blechschmidt's drawings (1963): epithelium was colored green, cartilage gray-blue, bone brown, and nerves yellow. In the present study arteries and veins were not distinguished by different colors: they were all painted red.

The reader may compare Fig 1g to Fig 59, and Fig 2 to Fig 11 to check the transition from contour-line plot to the anatomic drawing.

2.2.3 Graphic reconstruction compared to construction of solid models

Compared to the process of reconstructing a physical model, the computer-aided graphic reconstruction takes much less time. An important advantage of computer-aided three-dimensional reconstructions is the possibility of temporarily omitting certain structures, for example those which obscure the perspective view of more distinct structures.

A disadvantage, however, is the difficulty of obtaining metric data from a rotated graphic reconstruction. In addition, graphic reconstructions become more and more difficult to survey when the subjects become complex. Here the construction of solid models has a clear advantage but requires greater technical and time-consuming efforts.

The classical wax plate reconstruction technique was introduced by Born (1883, 1888). Here the contours were directly transferred to the wax plate, cut out, and composed as a reconstruction. Thickness of wax plates and magnification of the drawings on the wax plates must match each other. Wax, however, is not suffiently dimensionally stable (flowing under the pressure of the piled wax plates), and its stability is very dependent on a constant temperature. Reconstructions made from transparent materials like glass (Thomee 1928) or gelatine (Rolshoren 1937) are less easy for survey and are only suitable for smaller reconstructions. An improvement of the wax plate reconstruction was introduced by the casting mold technique *(Hohlgußverfahren)*, where the wax model serves only as a temporary mold, into which is poured a more stable material (Dankmeyer 1940). Blechschmidt (1954) developed a reconstruction technique using plastic resins, which allowed building of models about 1 m high. These reconstructions can still be observed in the embryological museum in the basement of the Institute of Anatomy of the University of Göttingen (Germany). Ooe (1956) produced his reconstruction models of tooth development from cardbord. Although today there are materials available that are easier to work with (for example, styrofoam plates), the construction of solid models still requires more of an effort than does a computer-graphic reconstruction. It is hoped that the computer-controlled industrial millingmachines will become available for research to produce embryological reconstruction models at low cost. Only then will computer-graphic reconstructions be replaced with solid reconstructions. Today computer-graphic reconstruction is still the method of choice.

3 Findings

All specimens listed in Table 1 have been reconstructed. In serial sections cut in a sagittal plane, both halves of the faces were reconstructed, but the description of the findings refers to the right half, because no principal differences were found between sides.

Some metric data are given in microns in the text. These data should be understood only as indications to facilitate perception of the spatial arrangement of the structures. The distances were obtained from nonrotated histologic sections and from calculations involving the thickness of the sections. These data should be understood in a qualitative sense rather than as statistically valid quantitative measurements. In addition, the usual changes of dimensions of the specimens due to chemical (fixation) and mechanical influences (the histologic processing techniques: embedding, cutting, stretching) must be considered concerning the validity of the measurements.

The reader will find characterizations of the primordia such as *round, oval, triangular, rectangular*. These terms should not be understood as purely geometric descriptions, but more as approximations. Findings of tooth development that are sufficently well known will not be repeated in detail; only such findings as are special and relevant for the question will be described.

The different tooth primordia are indicated with the usual letters: *i* for incisors, *c* for canines, and *m* for molars. Maxillary primordia are marked with superscript numbers, mandibular primordia with subscript numbers. (Although there is only one canine per quadrant in the human dentition, the number 1 has been used to denote the maxillary and mandibular canines by means of superscript and subscript ciphers, respectively.) Abbreviations used in the figures are based on the Nomina Anatomica conventions, and explanations are usually found in the legends.

As usual, *lateral* and *medial* refer to a displacement from the midline, whereas, as in dentistry, *distal* denotes the direction toward the end of the dental arch, and *mesial* to the midline. Because the dental arch describes a curve, *distal* and *lateral* are synonymous when used in reference to the anterior region of the dental arch, but in the molar region, *distal* indicates a posterior direction.

In order to facilitate comparison, all reconstructions (besides a few exceptions) are reproduced at the same magnification.

3.1 Stage of the dental lamina

The description of the morphology of the maxillary and the mandibular vestibular and dental lamina refers to the reconstruction of the embryo GUS (18 mm CRL). Prior to that is given a short description of the surrounding structures.

3.1.1 Maxillary region (Figs 2 and 4)

In this embryo GUS (18 mm CRL) the maxilla shows only a small extension. Branches of the maxillary nerve are not yet immured by bony structures. In the anterior region maxillary bone and dental lamina epithelium approach as close as 60 μm.

In this stage of development the vestibular lamina is not present continuously along the epithelial invagination. The dental lamina, in contrast, can be traced from the middle of the face in a lateral and distal direction, without interruption, for more than 2 mm. Its depth of invagination and its thickness is variable, so that its outline changes along the arch.

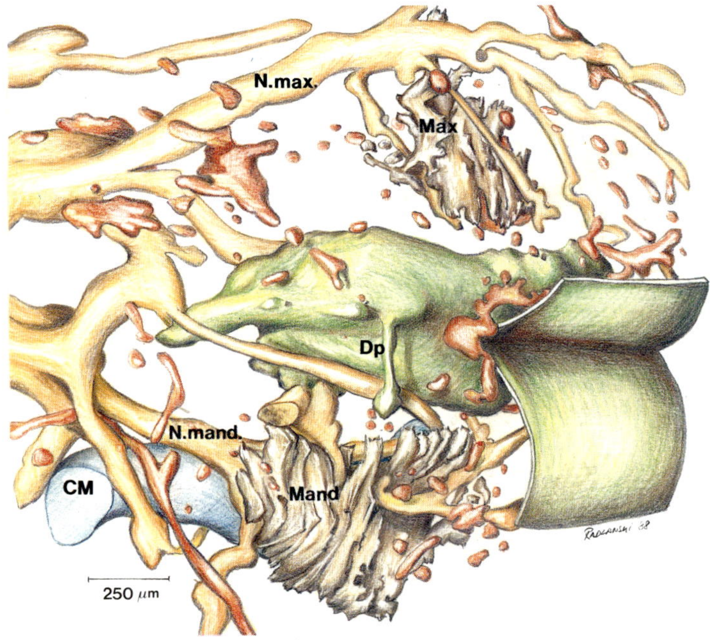

Fig 3 Embryo, 18 mm. Survey reconstruction of the right half of the oral cavity and its surrounding structures, lateral view, mesenchymal aspect of invaginated epithelium, painted green; parts of the upper and lower lip can be seen at the right margin of the figure. The dental primordia are in the lamina stage, hidden by the vestibular lamina (not labelled). The extension of the maxillary (Max) and the mandibular (Mand) bone, next to Meckel's cartilage (CM) is in an early stage. Branches of the innervation are already close to the oral epithelium. Some of the vessels are shown in the stage of single islands (which, however may be an artifact of reconstruction). (Dp) primordium of the parotid duct.

Both laminae, the dental and the vestibular, are clearly separated by a furrow that has varying depth and width along the arch. Also, both laminae arise from a common basal epithelial thickening in this region.

We will begin our more detailed description in the midfacial region and will follow the extension of the dental and vestibular laminae in a lateral direction. As an orientation in space, the distance from the middle of the face will be used, which is easy to determine because the thickness of sections is constantly 10 μm.

The epithelium covering the upper lip has an almost even thickness of 40 μm. In the midfacial region, toward the oral cavity, there is a fold of 130° in the surface of the epithelial covering. In the region of this fold, the epithelium is clearly thickened. Here it is invaginated into the mesenchyme for a depth of about 80 μm. The vestibular and dental lamina are separated by a just-visible, shallow furrow occupied by the mesenchyme.

In contrast to the midfacial region, where both laminae are invaginated to the same depth, at a point 60 μm more laterally, the vestibular lamina is invaginated almost twice as deep as the dental lamina. So in this region the separating furrow between the two laminae becomes more obvious. Further away from the midfacial region, at a distance of 120 μm, the depth of invagination of the vestibular lamina decreases again; here it is only one third deeper than the dental lamina. In this region both laminae are separated by a deep notch. Underneath this notch the epithelium is only 40 μm thick.

Further laterally, in the region between 240 μm and 750 μm from the middle of the face, the vestibular lamina is no longer present. In addition, in this region the fold of the epithelium toward the oral cavity is no longer as distinct as it was in the midfacial region. In sagittal section, the epithelial layer is evenly 60 μm thick; however, shortly before the invagination of the dental lamina, it is only about 40 μm thick. The dental lamina extends further laterally with a constant depth of invagination of about 160 μm, along a smooth curve in a dorsal direction. Its thickness in a vestibulo-oral direction decreases slightly.

At a distance of 750 μm away from the middle of

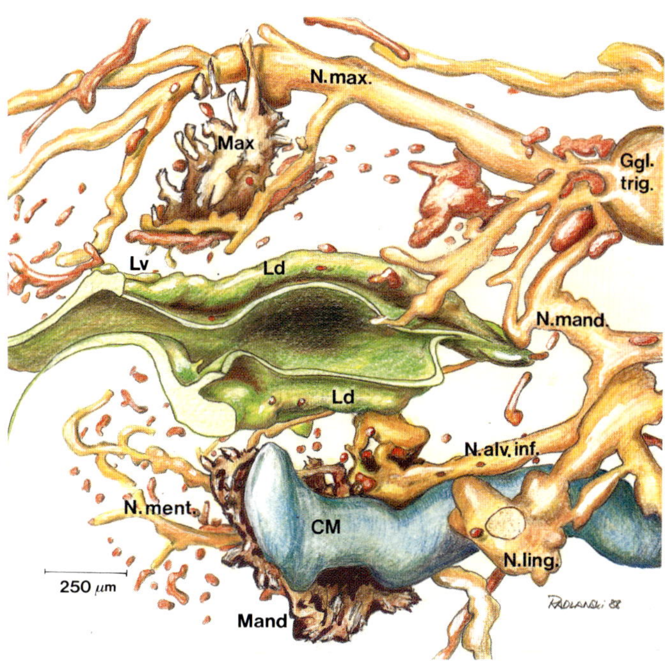

Fig 4 The same embryo (18 mm). Survey reconstruction of the right half of the oral cavity and its surrounding structures, medial view. Section plane at the left side of the figure is the midfacial sagittal plane. In the maxillary region the vestibular lamina (Lv) and the dental lamina (Ld) can be distinguished as two separate invaginations from a common epithelial protrusion. In the mandibular region the common invagination has not separated into a vestibular and a dental lamina towards the midfacial region; this separation is found only further laterally (not visible in the reconstruction). Medial to Meckel's cartilage there is no formation of mandibular bone (Mand). The mandibular structures obtain a retrognathic position toward the maxillary structures.

the face, the vestibular lamina, which had disappeared up to here, reappears. Lateral to the dental lamina there is a clearly visible thickening of the oral epithelium of 100 to 150 μm again. The dental lamina itself is stronger here: the furrow between the dental and the vestibular lamina is consequently more distinct.

The vestibular lamina of the maxillary region again recedes completely at about 1,200 μm lateral from the middle of the face. Here the oral epithelium is only 60 μm thick. The dental lamina can be traced further laterally. Several bulgings of 160 μm thickness are visible at first, before the normal thickness of the epithelium of 40 to 60 μm is reached 2,160 μm lateral to the middle of the face.

3.1.2 Mandibular region (Figs 3 to 5)

In the mandibular region, a bony plate forming the early mandible lies lateral and anterior to Meckel's cartilage. In the anterior region, close to the middle of the face, Meckel's cartilage rises above the bony plate for about 30 μm. Here the distance to the invaginated epithelial laminae is about 50 μm. At this stage the mandibular structures together obtain a retrognathic position toward the maxillary structures (Fig 4).

Whereas in the maxillary region the vestibular lamina was interrupted by leveling of the epithelium for a certain distance, it is more continuous in the mandibular region. However, a distinct separation between the vestibular and the dental lamina cannot be found continuously along the epithelial invagination. Thus, not every sagittal section taken from the midfacial region shows the furrow, which can be understood as the separation of the vestibular and dental laminae. (The shallow dent of the epithelial contour in the midfacial section in Fig 4 should not be interpreted as a separation between the two laminae, because it is located too far anteriorly.) The epithelial invaginations, which in this region represent the common vestibular and dental laminae, are more voluminous in contrast to that of the maxillary region. The depth of invagination is about 180 μm in the vertical and sagittal direction. Deeper, it is bent in a dorsal direction, and here the sagittal diameter is about 200 μm.

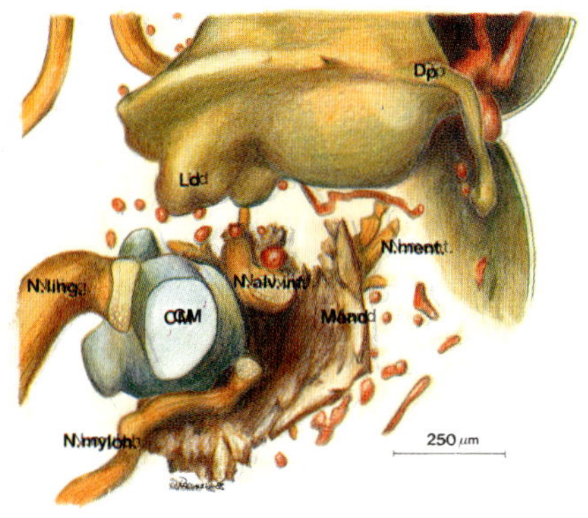

Fig 5 The same embryo (18 mm). Survey reconstruction of the dorsal aspect shows the spatial relationship between the epithelial formations of the dental lamina (Ld), Meckel's cartilage (CM), and the mandible (Mand) with the alveolar inferior nerve (N alv inf). In addition, lingual nerve (N ling), mylohyoid nerve (N myloh), and the primordium of the parotid duct (Dp) are labelled.

A little further laterally, 180 µm from the middle of the face, a shallow furrow in the epithelial invagination that separates the vestibular from the dental lamina can be seen. Further still (840 µm from the midfacial region) the depth of the epithelial invagination decreases gradually to about 100 µm, but it increases again to 150 µm at approximately 1,200 µm from the midfacial area.

In the lateral region of the epithelial arch (1,140 to 1,500 µm from midface), the separation of dental and vestibular laminae is very clearly marked. Both laminae are invaginated to about the same depth, separated by a groove of the same depth. At a distance of 1,920 µm from the middle of the face, the epithelial invagination levels out to the normal thickness of 40 µm.

3.2 Bud stage

3.2.1 Early bud stage

The description of this stage refers to the reconstruction of the embryo ALI (21 mm CRL).

3.2.1.1 Maxillary region (Fig 6)

At regular intervals of about 425 µm (measured edge-to-edge), the dental lamina shows knoblike swellings that are called the *tooth buds*. In horizontal section, these buds are almost round in the maxillary region, and they are approximately 200 µm in diameter. The primordia i^1 and i^2, and c^1 are clearly recognizable in the reconstruction. Although the molar primordia are discernible in the histologic sections, their protrusions do not show up clearly in the reconstruction: the posterior region of the dental and vestibular laminae is characterized by an abundance of irregular foldings and epithelial protrusions.

In the tooth buds, the marginal epithelial cells assume a wedge-shaped outline at the bulgings (Fig 8). In the areas between the tooth buds, the cells of the dental lamina obtain a more cuboid outline.

The distance between the tooth buds and the bony structures of the early maxilla is about 60 to 80 µm. In a distal direction, the ascending part of the maxilla confines the posterior space for expansion of the epithelium and comes as close as 400 µm. Meckel's cartilage, which runs medially from the mandibular bone, comes as close as 550 to 600 µm from the maxillary epithelial formations from dorsal direction.

The mesenchyme is condensed around every tooth primordium.

3.2.1.2 Mandibular region (Fig 7)

The tooth buds arise at the lingual side of the invaginated epithelium as prominent protrusions. The distance separating the tooth buds in the mandibular dental lamina is 250 to 300 µm and so is less than that in the maxillary lamina; the primordia of i_1, however, are even closer together, being separated by a distance of only 170 µm.

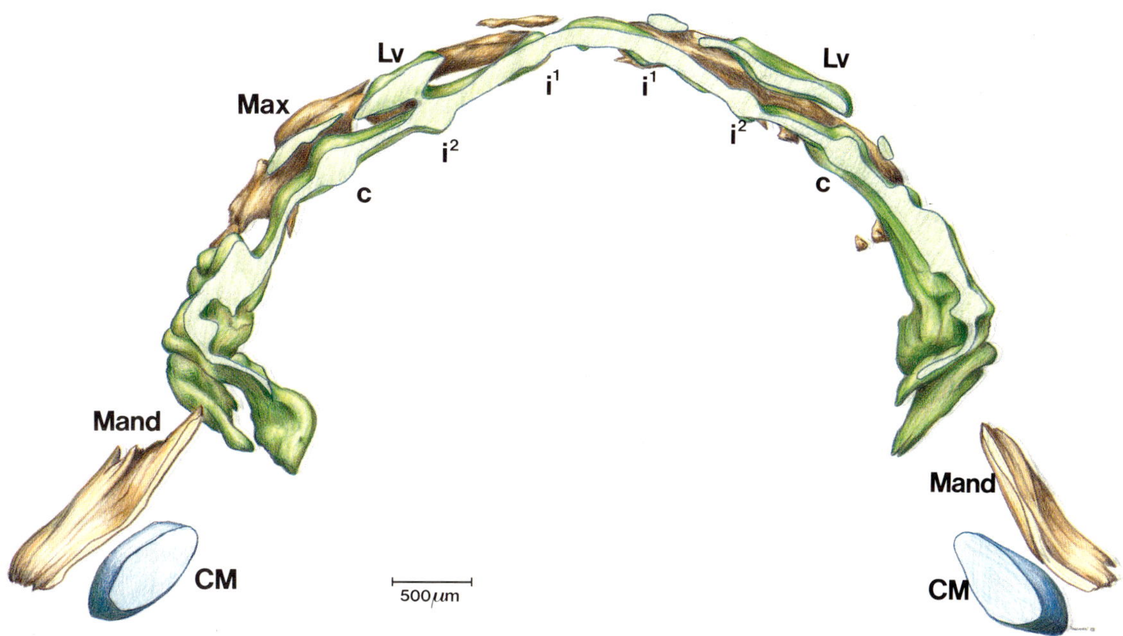

Fig 6 Embryo, 21 mm. Reconstruction of the maxilla, caudal aspect, to show the spatial relationship between the dental lamina, the vestibular lamina (Lv), parts of maxillary (Max) and mandibular (Mand) bone, and Meckel's cartilage (CM). The dental primordia i^1, i^2 and c are in their bud stage.

While the buds in the maxillary dental lamina are almost round, the buds of i_1 are clearly flat. Their extension in the vestibulo-oral direction is only 125 μm, while their mesiodistal dimension is about 250 μm. The bud i_2 is not quite round in this stage and has a diameter of about 170 μm; c_1 is rounder and larger, with a diameter of about 250 μm. The primordia m_1 and m_2 have an almost oval form and are of quite the same size; their mesiodistal diameter is approximately 360 μm, and their transverse diameter about 160 μm.

The vestibular lamina extends distally only as far as the region of the primordium of the first molar. Here it is located further laterally than in the anterior region, where it runs closer to the dental lamina.

As in the maxillary region, the mandibular mesenchyme is condensed around each tooth bud.

The spatial relations of the invaginated epithelium to the mandible and to Meckel's cartilage are represented in Fig 7. The space for a possible dorsal extension of the epithelium is limited by the ascending parts of the mandible and Meckel's cartilage. In the anterior region Meckel's cartilage comes as close as 130 μm to the buds of i_1 lingually. However, it lies further away from the round buds of i_2. The greatest distance from Meckel's cartilage is found with c_1: here there exist bony structures between the bud and cartilage. Further distally, Meckel's cartilage and the dental epithelium approach, because here the cartilaginous bar bends upward in a dorsal direction, and the dental lamina bends medially in the vicinity of the ascendent ramus of the mandible. The distance between the primordium m_2 and the mandibular bone is about 300 μm in this region.

3.2.2 Late bud stage

No illustrations are presented for this embryo (OLL, 28 mm CRL), but a brief description will be added

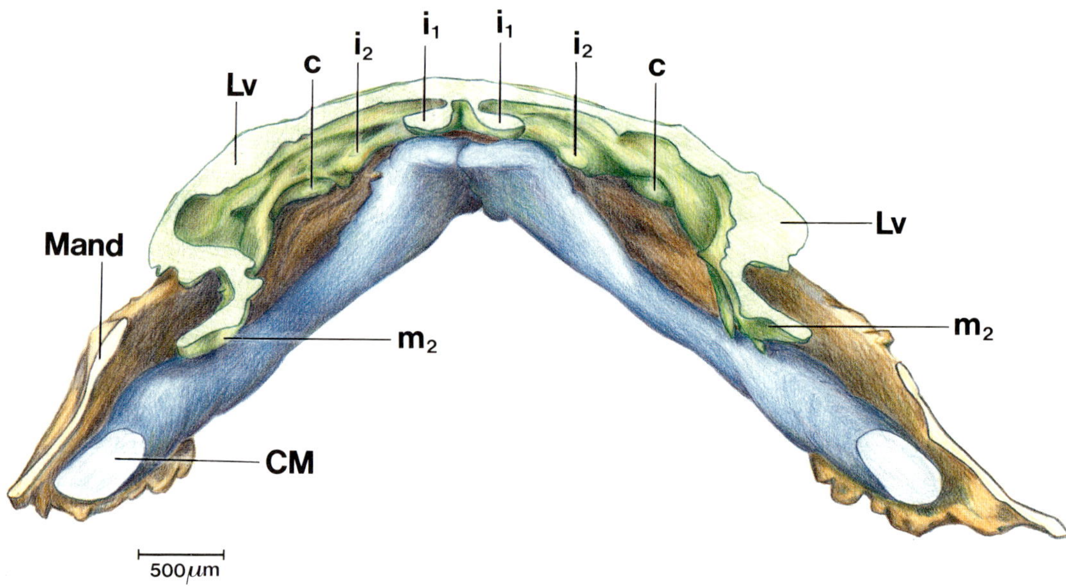

Fig 7 The same embryo (21 mm). Reconstruction of the mandible, cranial aspect, shows the spatial relationship between the dental lamina, the vestibular lamina (Lv), mandibular bone (Mand), and Meckel's cartilage (CM). The dental primordia i_1, i_2, c, m_1 and m_2 are in their bud stage, but m_1 is hidden by protruding epithelial foldings.

to the description of the findings of the early bud stage.

In the maxillary midfacial region, the furrow between the vestibular lamina and the dental lamina is very shallow. Further laterally, but before the bud of i^1 is reached, it becomes increasingly deeper. The bud i^1 is well rounded, with a clearly visible enamel knot (Ahrens 1913a) that protrudes as a lens-shaped formation from the bud. The bud i^2 is visible only as a slight thickening of the dental lamina cranially. The primordium of c^1 is present as a bud that is not quite round, being slightly flattened in a cranial direction. The primordial region of m^1 is discernible as a flat but extended protrusion of the dental lamina, while the primordium of m^2 can be realized only as a slight protrusion of the lateral oral epithelium.

In the mandibular midfacial region the furrow between the dental and vestibular laminae is as shallow as described for the maxillary region. It becomes very distinct only in the region of the primordium of i_1. This bud is flat and oval, with its mesiodistal and cranio-caudal extensions greater than those in vestibulo-oral direction. The primordium of i_2 shows characteristics similar to those of i_1. The same pattern of flattening is present, but is less imposing because of the overal' smaller size of the bud. The primordium of c_1 has already reached the cap stage and reaches beyond the vestibular lamina almost twice as far as its invaginated depth. The primordium of m_1 has also attained the cap stage and is already slightly oval, with its greatest diamter in the direction of the dental lamina arch. The m_2 bud is discernible as a little oval protrusion 50 μm from the distal end of the dental lamina.

3.3 Bud and early cap stage

The description of this stage refers to the reconstruction of the fetus DOR (37 mm CRL), in which most of the primordia resemble the stage of buds and early caps.

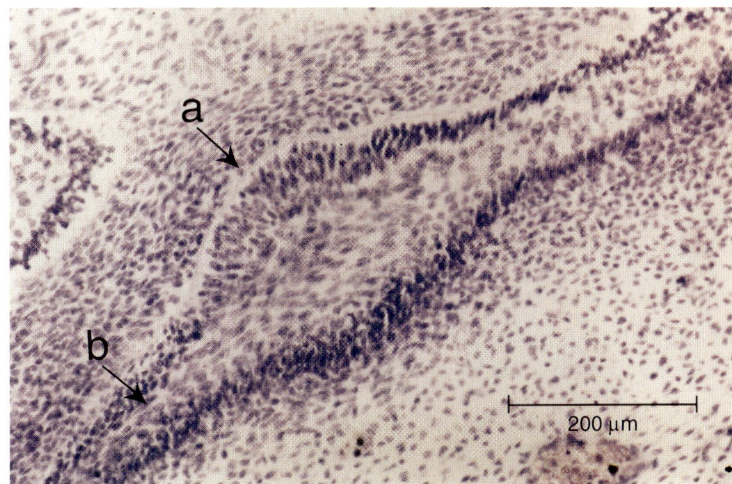

Fig 8 Embryo, 21 mm. Horizontal section through the dental primordium of c[1] in the bud stage. In the buds the marginal epithelial cells have a predominantly wedged shape (a), whereas in the dental lamina area between the buds the marginal epithelial cells are more cuboid (b).

3.3.1 Primordium of i[1] (Figs 10 and 12)

The tooth primordium of i[1] has reached the typical bud stage: the protrusion of the epithelium is almost completely round and the enamel knot is markedly developed. Between the dental lamina and the vestibular lamina runs a deep furrow that clearly separates the two epithelial invaginations. At the labial aspect of the vestibular lamina, in the region of the primordium i[1], there is an additional folding of the invaginated epithelium (Figs 12 and 13). It has a transverse extension of about 60 μm. (A similar finding was recorded in the fetus ILO, 40 mm CRL, but here the extension ran for about 200 μm.)

The maxillary bony structures in this region extend as close as 100 μm toward the epithelium of the vestibular and dental laminae.

3.3.2 Primordium of i[2] (Figs 10 and 14)

The bud of i[2] is smaller than that of i[1]. The vestibular lamina is slightly bulged mesially and distally from the bud. The distance between the vestibular lamina and the primordium of the second incisor is slightly greater than that between the lamina and the primordium of the first incisor.

The maxilla, which reaches down as close as 90 μm toward the epithelial formations, forms a groove in this region that is open orally. In this groove the superior alveolar nerve and its accompanying blood vessels can be found.

3.3.3 Primordium of c[1] (Figs 15 to 18)

The primordium of c[1] has already reached the cap stage, with its vestibular and oral margins slightly protruded. The mesial margin is less bulged. Although slight bulging of the distal margin is also present, it appears less prominent because the complete primordium is tilted in a distal direction. A lateral enamel lamina (Bolk 1913) and consequently a distal enamel niche (Bolk 1913) are clearly developed (Figs 17 and 18). When looked upon from a cranial direction, the outline of the cap resembles a triangle in which one tip points distally. Mesially from the primordium of c[1], some parts of the maxilla extend down into the wide furrow between vestibular and dental laminae (Fig 15), while distally they reach a distance of more than 200 μm (Fig 17).

3.3.4 Primordium of m[1] (Figs 9 and 19)

The primordium of m[1] has reached the early cap stage. It has an angular outline and is bent distally.

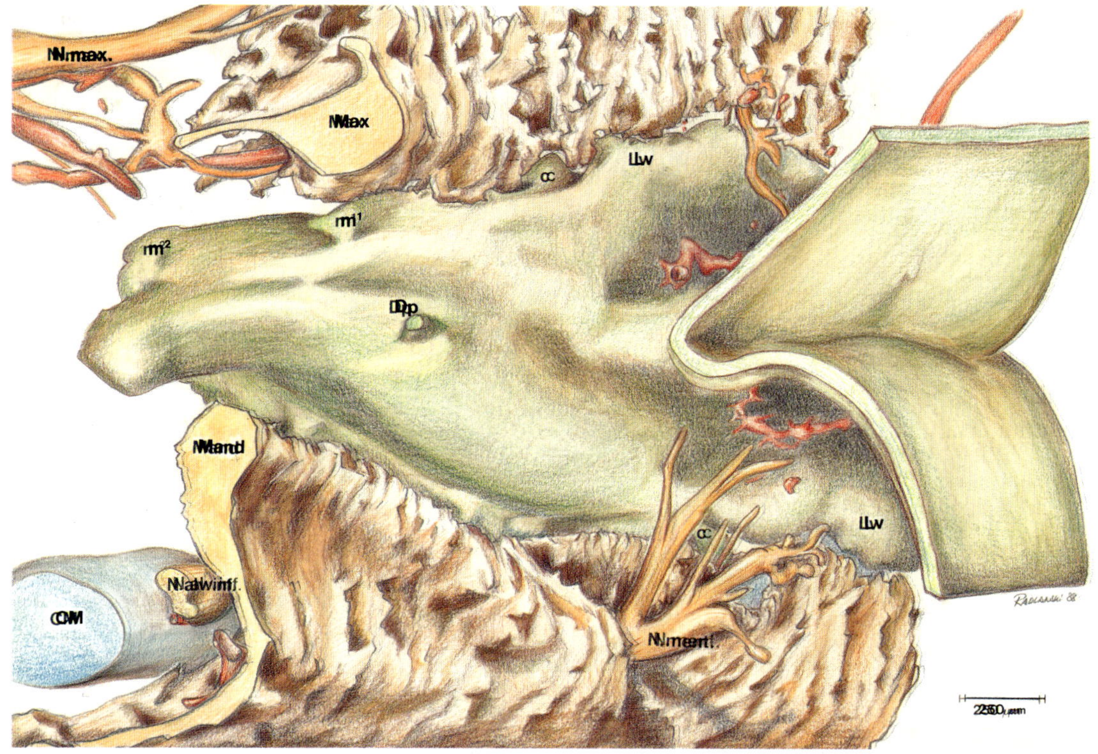

Fig 9 Fetus, 37 mm. Survey reconstruction of the right half of the oral cavity and its surrounding structures, lateral view, mesenchymal aspect of invaginated epithelium (green). Parts of the upper and lower lip at the right margin of the picture. In the maxillary region the vestibular lamina (Lv) covers the dental primordia of the anterior teeth, whereas the canine and molar primordia are visible. Extensions of the maxillary bone (Max) reach down closely to the oral epithelium and the primordia, except for m^2. In the mandibular region all primordia except c are covered by mandibular bone (Mand). Meckel's cartilage (CM, blue) protrudes into the anterior region between vestibular lamina (Lv) and the incisor primordia (hidden). The mental foramen (at N ment) opens slightly distal of the primordium of c_1. The parotid duct (cut, Dp) has become displaced distally, compared to the situation in the 18-mm embryo (Fig 3).

The maxilla lies 100 μm cranial to the primordium, while it descends closer to the dental lamina in the region between the primordia m^1 and c^1.

3.3.5 Primordium of m^2 (Figs 9 and 19)

The most distal epithelium of the dental lamina protrudes to form a bud, the primordium of m^2, which is clearly bent in a distal direction. In contrast to the other primordia of this stage, the maxilla is particularly far away from the bud: directly cranially there is no bone, and in an anterior direction, there runs an extension of the maxilla in a distance of about 250 μm (Fig 19).

3.3.6 Primordium of i_1 (Figs 19 to 21)

The primordium of i_1 represents the stage of an early cap. Marginal bulgings are present but very weakly developed. The mesiodistal diameter is approximately 200 μm, and it is greater than its vestibulo-oral diameter, which is only about 160 μm.

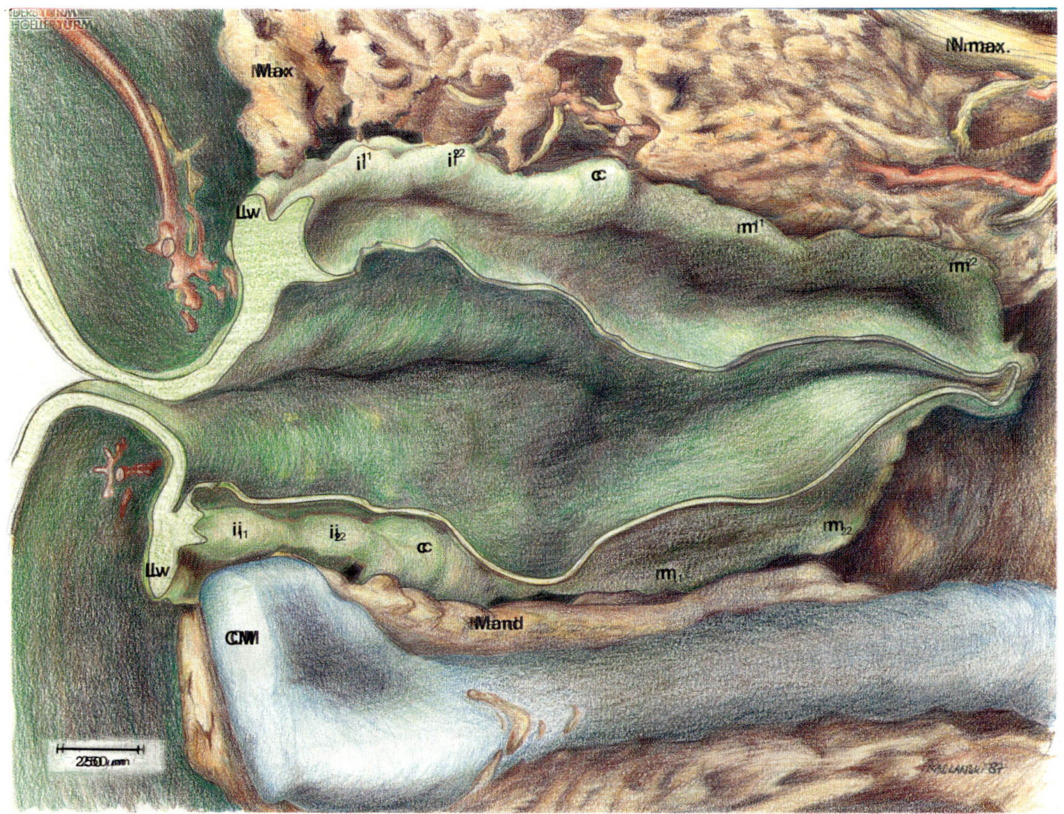

Fig 10 The same fetus (37 mm). Survey reconstruction of the right half of the oral cavity and its surrounding structures, medial view. Plane of section is the midfacial plane. At the left margin the contours of upper and lower lip, which merge into the epithelial invaginations of the vestibular lamina (Lv). The dental primordia i^1, i^2, and m^2 have reached the bud stage, the primordia c^1 and m^1 are in the early cap stage. Extensions of the maxilla (Max) reach down into the furrow between the dental and the vestibular lamina (Lv). In the mandibular arch, i_2 and m_2 are in their bud stage, and the primordia i_1, c_1, and m_1 have reached the early cap stage. Meckel's cartilage (CM) protrudes close to the bud i_1, between the other primordia and Meckel's cartilage there arise parts of mandibular bone (Mand). In contrast to the situation in the 18-mm fetus (Fig 4), the mandible obtains a mesial relation to the maxillary structures.

In a caudal direction, the vestibular lamina invaginates further down than the tooth primordium, which diverges from the common epithelial invagination at about half the depth, and extends more horizontally in an oral direction. The epithelial cells in the cap are more densely packed than the cells that form the vestibular lamina. Superior to the cap i_1, toward the oral cavity, the invaginated epithelium folds to form a minor additional lamina, which arises more medially but levels out toward the middle of the primordium. The most anterior flattened part of Meckel's cartilage arises from a caudal direction and approaches as close as 40 μm to the primordium. The mesenchyme around the cap is very clearly condensed. Within the cartilage, most of the cells are swollen, thus indicating growth-extension of the cartilaginous structure. The mesenchymal cells surrounding the anterior end of Meckel's cartilage have an elongated form and are arranged like the waves in front of a moving ship (Fig 21). In the region anterior to Meckel's cartilage, a flat extension of mandibular bone has formed.

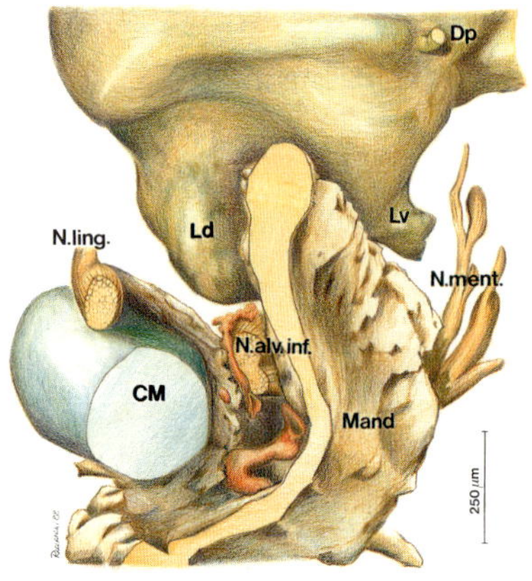

Fig 11 The same fetus (37 mm). Survey reconstruction, dorsal view, illustrates the spatial relationship between the epithelial invaginations of the dental lamina (Ld), vestibular lamina (Lv), mandible (Mand), Meckel's cartilage (CM), and the alveolar inferior (N alv inf), the mental (N ment), and the lingual nerve (N ling). Red indicates inferior alveolar artery and vein. (Dp) parotid duct, cut.

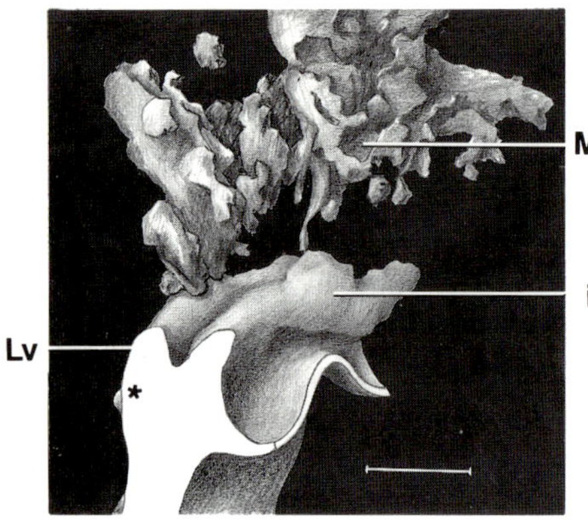

Fig 12 The same fetus (37 mm). Partial reconstruction illustrates the right bud i^1, the vestibular lamina (Lv), and the maxilla (Max), medial view. Left of the area marked by the asterisk is an additional folding of the vestibular lamina (compare Fig 13). Scale: 250 μm.

3.3.7 Primordium of i_2 (Figs 10 and 22)

The primordium of i_2 has reached the early cap stage, and marginal bulgings are, like the primordium of i_1, only very weakly developed. The primordium of the second incisor has about the same size and oval form as the primordium of the central incisor, described above. The flat, anterior part of Meckel's cartilage comes as close as 35 μm to the dental lamina mesially from the primordium. Then, however, before the protrusion of the primordium is reached, the flat part of Meckel's cartilage ends, and its contour descends steeply in a caudal and posterior direction. This region of Meckel's cartilage is covered by mandibular bone, which arises laterally between the tooth primordium and cartilage. The distance between the cap i_2 and the mandible is different mesially and distally because the mandibular bone descends obliquely more and more distally. Therefore, mesially the distance between primordium and bone is about 60 μm, while distally it is more than 100 μm. Further distally the mandible gradually forms a groove into which the primordium of the canine descends.

3.3.8 Primordium of c_1 (Figs 23 and 24)

The primordium c_1 reaches further caudally than the vestibular lamina in this region. This canine primordium has clearly attained the cap stage, with a circular marginal bulging. In this way, what will eventually become the inner enamel epithelium displays a shallow trough toward the underlying

Fig 13a Sagittal section of the maxillary laminar region of the same fetus (37 mm), medial of the right primordium i^1. Anterior to the vestibular lamina (Lv) lies the additional invagination of the epithelium. (Ld) dental lamina.

Fig 13b Reconstruction of the vestibular lamina (Lv) in the i^1 region and mesial thereof of the same 37-mm fetus. Anterior view, 20° lateral and 20° cranial. From this reconstruction it becomes obvious that the additional invagination is a folding of the vestibular lamina. Next to the asterisk lies the plane of section of Fig 13a. In addition, the invaginational depth is less in medial direction for about 150 μm. (Ld) dental lamina. Scale: 250 μm.

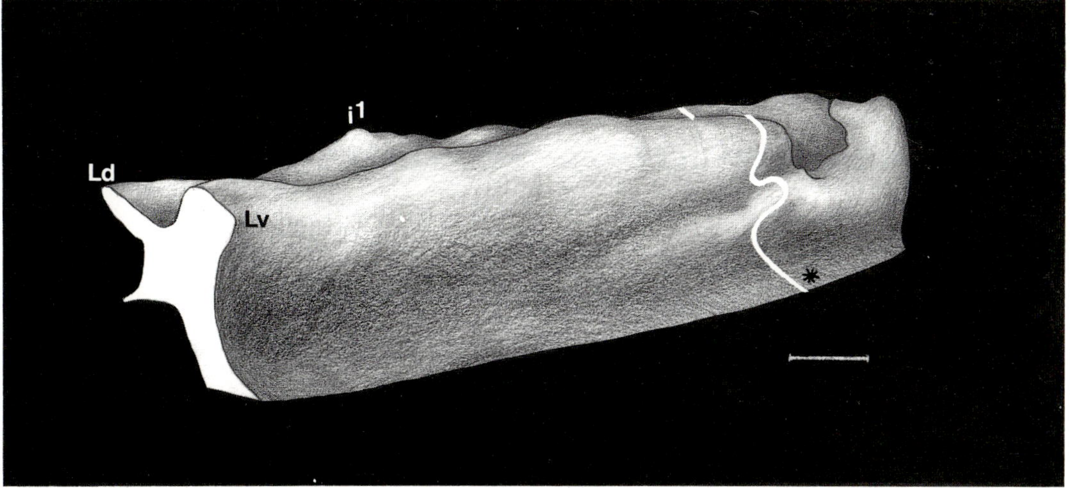

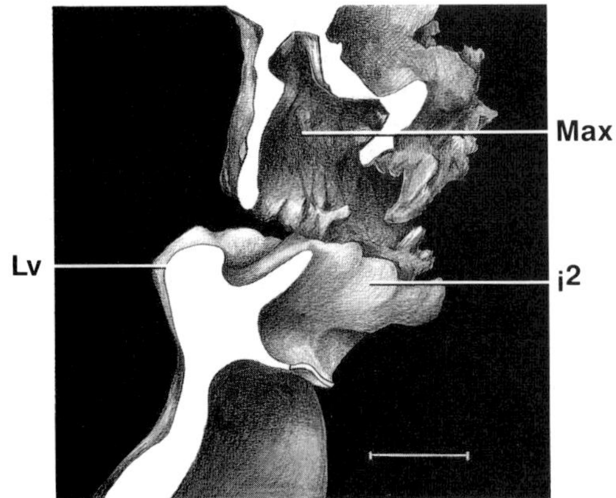

Fig 14 The same fetus (37 mm). Partial reconstruction illustrates the right bud i^2, the vestibular lamina (Lv), and the maxilla (Max). Medial view. Scale: 250 μm.

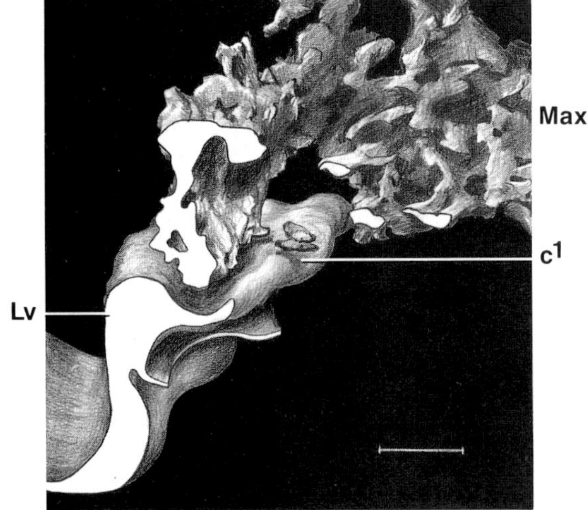

Fig 15 The same fetus (37 mm). Partial reconstruction illustrates the right bud c^1, the vestibular lamina (Lv), and the maxilla (Max). Medial view. Scale: 250 μm.

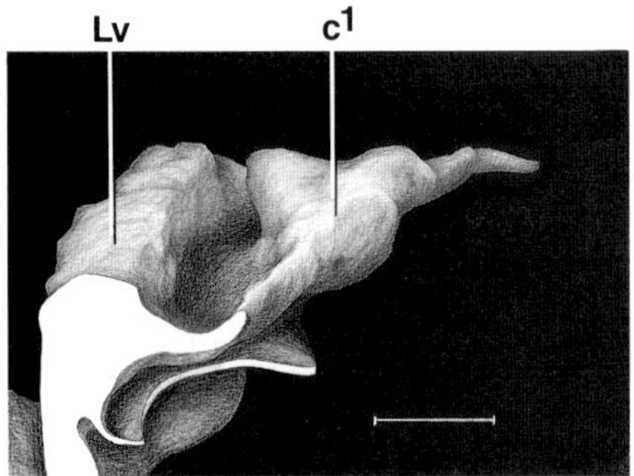

Fig 16 The same fetus (37 mm). Partial reconstruction illustrates the right bud c^1 and the vestibular lamina (Lv) in a medial view, but without covering maxilla. Scale: 250 μm.

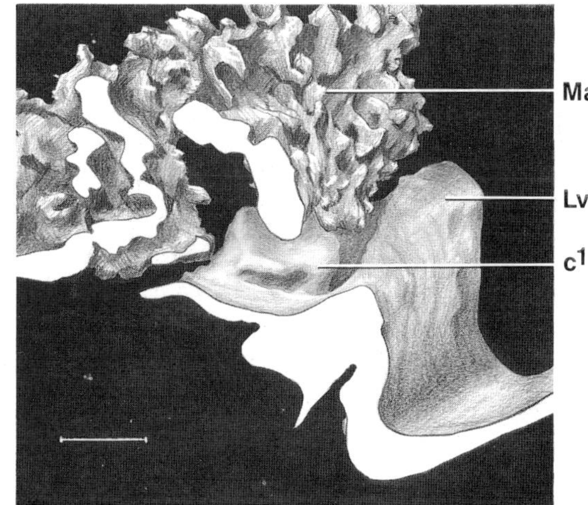

Fig 17 The same fetus (37 mm). Partial reconstruction illustrates the right bud c^1, the vestibular lamina (Lv), and the maxilla (Max). Lateral view. Scale: 250 μm.

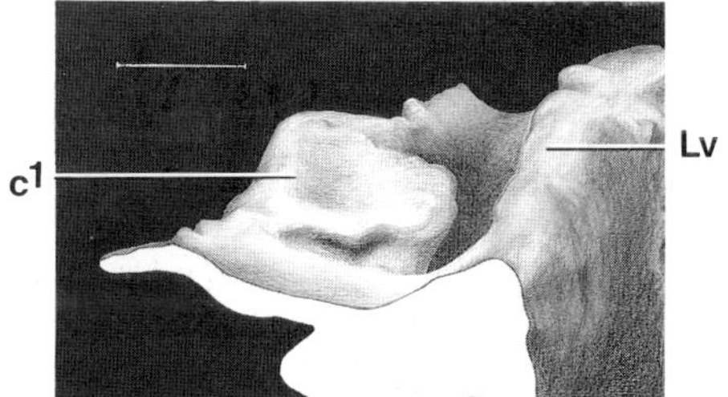

Fig 18 The same fetus (37 mm). Partial reconstruction illustrates the right bud c^1 and the vestibular lamina (Lv) in a lateral view, but without covering maxilla. Scale: 250 μm.

mandible. The cap is tilted distally, and a lateral enamel lamina (Bolk 1913) and an enamel niche, pointing distally, is well developed here, as it is in the maxillary arch. In an occlusal view (ie, seen from a vertical perspective), the outline of the primordium c_1 is rather round, as compared to that of the maxillary canine primordium, which was more triangular in shape.

The primordium c_1 has no contact with Meckel's cartilage because it is located too far laterally from this structure. Beneath the primordium, the mandible has formed a groove into which the primordium descends from a medial direction. From a distal direction, however, there arises a thin bony plate that partly covers the bony groove and comes as close as about 35 μm to the primordium of c_1. No increased number of osteoclasts was observed in this specific region.

3.3.9 Primordium of m_1 (Fig 25)

The primordium of the first primary mandibular molar has reached the late cap stage, with many voluminous marginal bulgings, of which the mesial, and particularly the distal, are lower. The primordium is extended in a mesiodistal direction. The vestibular lamina is located laterally from the dental lamina as a separate invagination of the oral

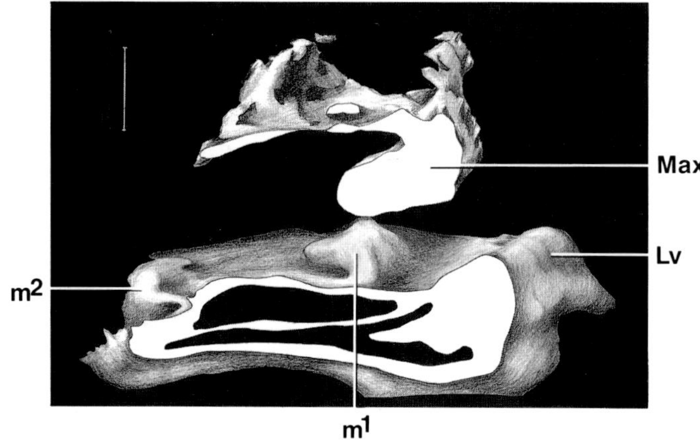

Fig 19 The same fetus (37 mm). Partial reconstruction illustrates the right cap m^1 and the bud m^2, the vestibular lamina (Lv), and the maxilla (Max). Lateral view. The small triangle denotes the cut surface of the mesenchyme, which is cranial of the oral cavity. This cut surface is due to the wide medial extension of the dental epithelium. Scale: 250 μm.

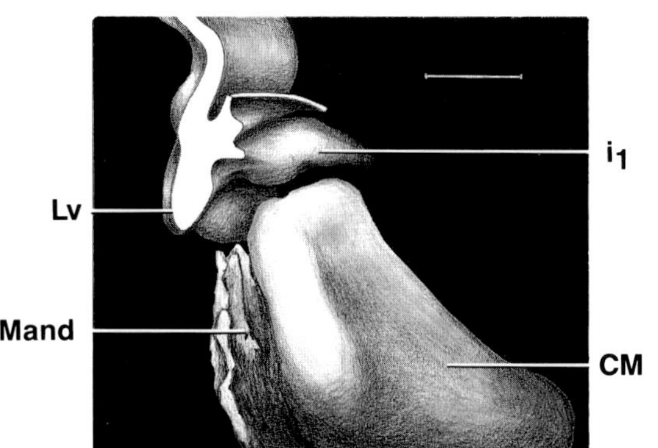

Fig 20 The same fetus (37 mm). Partial reconstruction illustrates the right cap i_1, the vestibular lamina (Lv), Meckel's cartilage (CM) and the mandible (Mand). Medial view. Scale: 250 μm.

epithelium, and, coming from mesial direction, before it reaches the region of the molar's primordium, it recedes.

The primordium of the first primary molar is located above of the large, v-shaped groove that has formed in the mandible. The margins of this bony groove are found no closer than 200 to 300 μm from the primordium. In the center of this groove run the inferior alveolar nerve and the homonymous artery; the inferior alveolar vein courses along the bottom of the groove. The bony groove has a maximal width of about 450 to 500 μm in the region of m_1 but narrows further distally, as depicted in Fig 11.

3.3.10 Primordium of m_2 (Fig 25)

The distal end of the dental lamina is swollen and gives rise to a bud that is the primordium of m_2. Mandibular bone is about 310 μm away laterally, and Meckel's cartilage lies medially, about 340 μm away.

3.4 Cap stage

The description of this stage refers to the reconstructions of the fetus NIN (47 mm CRL).

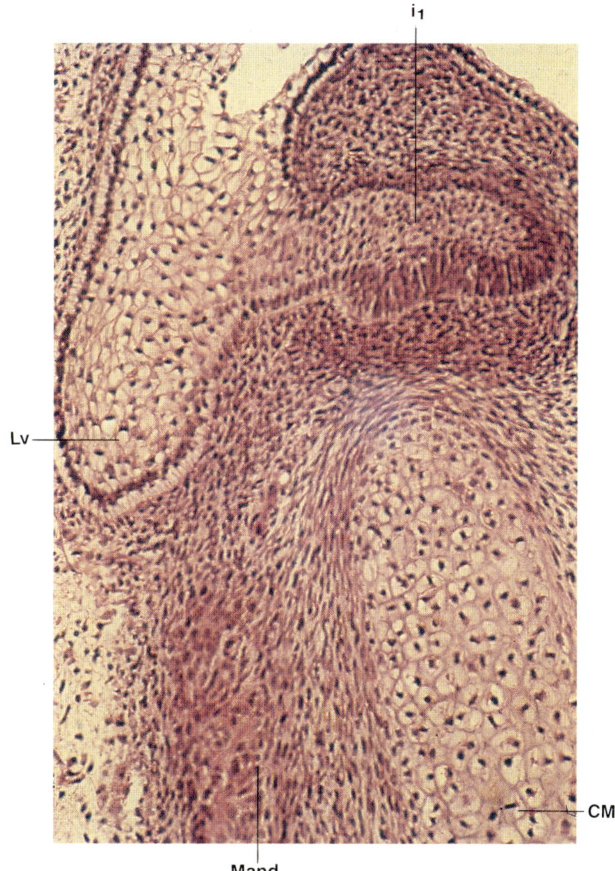

Fig 21 Sagittal section through the early cap i_1 of the same fetus (37 mm). The bubbly chondrocytes of Meckel's cartilage (CM) indicate its extension, and the surrounding mesenchymal cells are clearly condensed predominantly cranial of CM. The epithelium of the bud itself is more condensed than that of the vestibular lamina (Lv).

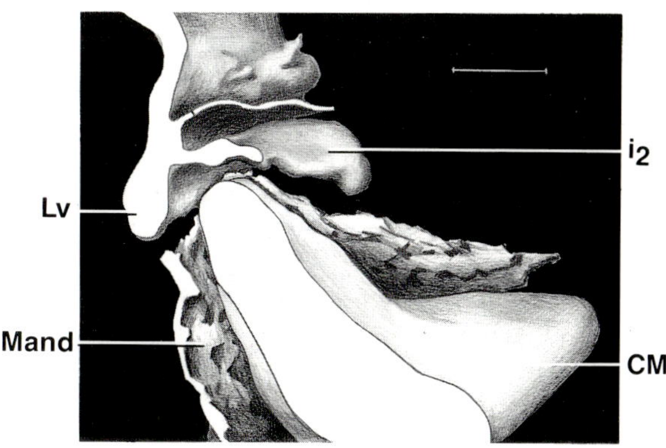

Fig 22 The same fetus (37 mm). Partial reconstruction illustrates the right cap i_2, the vestibular lamina (Lv), Meckel's cartilage (CM), and the mandible (Mand). Medial view. Scale: 250 μm.

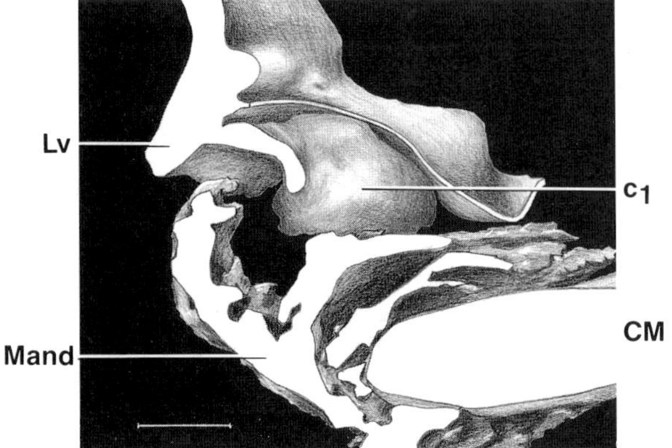

Fig 23 The same fetus 37 mm. Partial reconstruction illustrates the right cap c_1, the vestibular lamina (Lv), Meckel's cartilage (CM), and the mandible (Mand). Medial view. Scale: 250 μm.

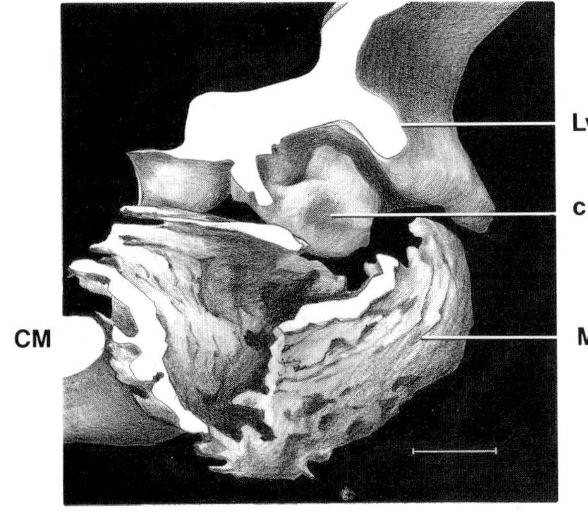

Fig 24 The same fetus (37 mm). Partial reconstruction illustrates the right cap c_1, the vestibular lamina (Lv), Meckel's cartilage (CM), and the mandible (Mand). Lateral view. Scale: 250 μm.

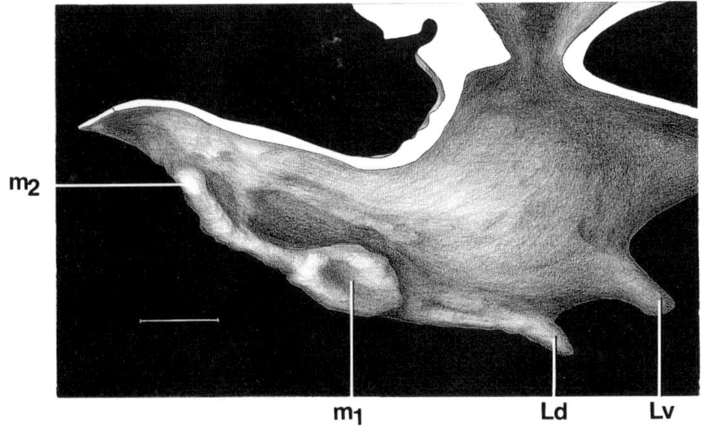

Fig 25 The same fetus (37 mm). Partial reconstruction illustrates the right bud m_2, the cap m_1, the dental lamina (Ld), and the vestibular lamina (Lv) in a lateral view. Scale: 250 μm.

Fig 26a Fetus, 47 mm. Partial reconstruction, in a medial view, illustrates the spatial relationship between the right cap i^1, parts of the vestibular lamina (Lv), the maxilla (Max), and the nerves and vessels, which run in the bony groove. Scale: 250 μm.

Fig 26b Lateral view of the same reconstruction. Scale: 250 μm.

Fig 27a The same fetus (47 mm). Partial reconstruction, medial view, illustrates the spatial relationship between the right cap i^2, the vestibular lamina (Lv), the maxilla (Max), and the nerves and vessels. Scale: 250 μm.

Fig 27b Lateral view of the same reconstruction. Scale: 250 μm.

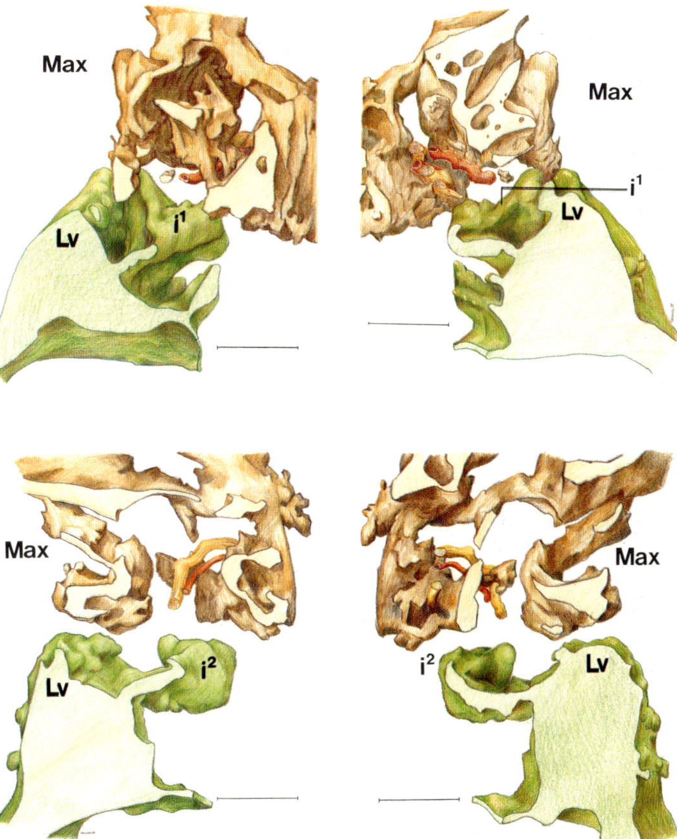

3.4.1 Primordium of i^1 (Figs 26 and 35)

The primordium of i^1 has reached the typical cap stage in this fetus. The circular bulge of this cap is well developed. It is, however, slightly irregular in thickness, and decends further mesially than distally. The lateral enamel lamina (Bolk 1913) is developed as a strong stem, and the enamel niche (Bolk 1913) has developed as a deep funnel distally. In a mesial direction, only a slight hint of an enamel trough (Meyer 1951) is recognizable because the marginal bulge of the cap is somewhat prominent here. There is no deep excavation toward the lateral enamel lamina (Bolk 1913). The enamel knot (Ahrens 1913a) is well developed.
In contrast to the incisor primordia of a younger fetus in earlier stages, in this fetus the cap of i^1 is clearly flat; its mesiodistal direction is much greater than its vestibulo-oral diameter. Accordingly, the enamel knot is no longer well rounded but matches the clearly marked mesiodistal flattening of the cap. The cap i^1 has a vestibular protrusion of its circular bulge rising slightly above the vestibular lamina.
The epithelial cap of i^1 is surrounded by a bony crypt, which, next to the cap, contains the adjacent surrounding mesenchyme. There are some medial and lateral, as well as oral and vestibular, extensions of the maxillary bone that come closer to the epithelial formations. A vestibular bony extension reaches deep into the sulcus between the tooth primordium and the vestibular lamina and comes as close as 100 μm (Fig 26a). In the bony crypt the superior alveolar artery, vein, and nerve can be seen.

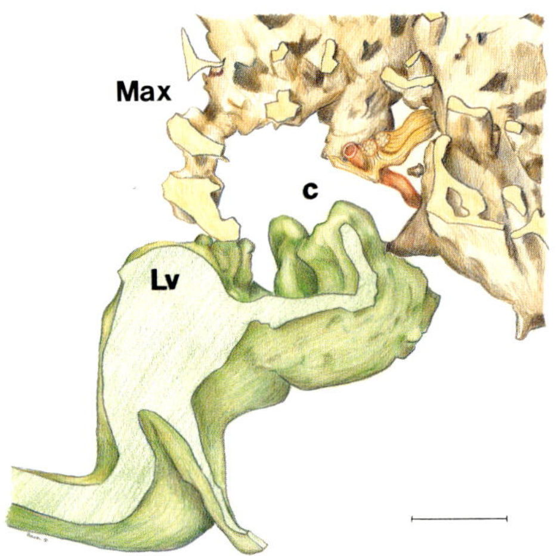

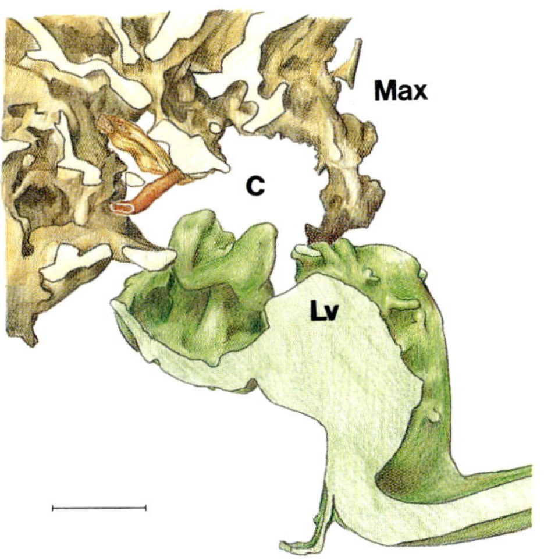

Fig 28 a The same fetus (47 mm). Partial reconstruction, medial view, illustrates the spatial relationship between the right cap c^1, the vestibular lamina (Lv), the maxilla (Max), and the nerves and vessels. Scale: 250 μm.

Fig 28 b Lateral view of the same reconstruction. Scale: 250 μm.

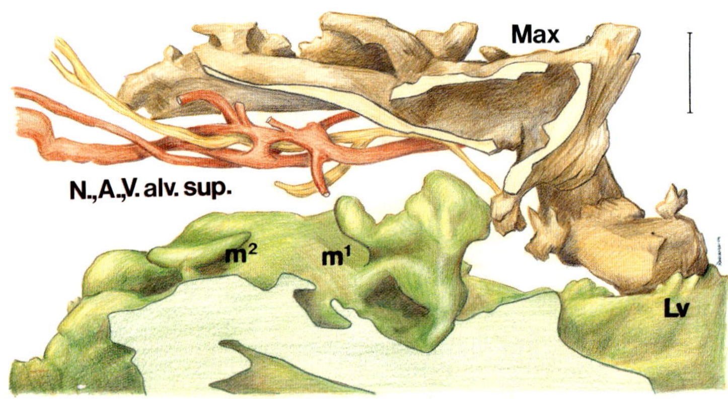

Fig 29 The same fetus (47 mm). Partial reconstruction, illustrates the spatial relationship between the right caps m^1 and m^2, the vestibular lamina (Lv), the maxilla (Max), and the nerves and vessels (N, A, V alv sup) in a lateral view. Scale: 250 μm.

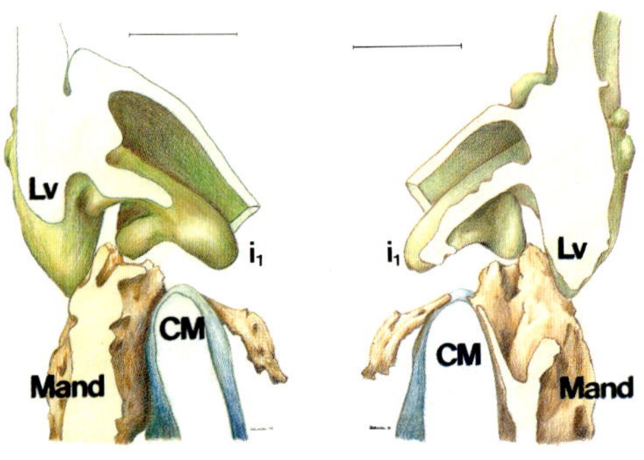

Fig 30 a The same fetus (47 mm). Partial reconstruction illustrates the spatial relationship between the right cap i_1, the vestibular lamina (Lv), Meckel's cartilage (CM), and the mandible (Mand) in a medial view. Scale: 250 μm.

Fig 30 b The same reconstruction, shown in a lateral view. Scale: 250 μm.

3.4.2 Primordium of i^2 (Figs 27 and 36)

The cap i^2 is smaller than the primordium of the maxillary central incisor. Consequently, the lateral enamel lamina is smaller, and the enamel knot protrudes only slightly. The form of the cap shows a greater extension in a mesio-distal direction, and, whereas its mesial contour is rounded, its distal margin is more acute. Further, the bulging of the distal margin is slightly thinner than the mesial margin. The distance between the primordium i^2 and the vestibular lamina is almost twice as great as it is in the region of i^1. Distally a clearly visible enamel niche has formed, whereas mesially there is no enamel trough.
Extensions of the maxillary bone come as close as 30 μm to the vestibular lamina, while they maintain a minimal distance of 70 μm to the cap i^2. Cranial to i^2, there is an area free of bone that corresponds to the layer of condensed mesenchyme around the cap.

3.4.3 Primordium of c^1 (Figs 28 and 37)

There are particular differences between the primordium of the canine and the incisor primordia described above. Besides the overall form, these differences are due to the expression of the marginal bulging and the tilting of the cap. The circular bulge is markedly thinner mesially and distally, while it is thicker on the palatal and vestibular margins. In addition, the cap c^1 seems to be tilted distally, so that its margin here runs much closer to the epithelium of the dental lamina. Toward the vestibular lamina, the marginal bulging of the cap becomes much thicker and extends into the lateral enamel lamina with almost no change in thickness. Thus, mesially (Fig 28a) a deep enamel niche is formed. Distally a larger enamel niche is formed, containing a secondary lamina (Fig 28b). The cap c^1 has an almost triangular shape if seen from an oblique cranial direction (Fig 37), with one tip of the triangle pointing into the direction of the vestibular lamina. The enamel knot is clearly visible but is atypically divided by a furrow that runs in a mesiodistal direction.
Extensions of the maxillary bone reach down to the vestibular lamina as close as 50 μm, whereas they do not come closer than 60 μm to the cap i^1. As noted above for the incisor caps, there is a bone-free region corresponding to the condensed mesenchyme surrounding the epithelial structures of the primordium. In the depth of this bony crypt the superior alveolar artery, vein, and nerve can be seen (Fig 28). In this region the common invagination of the oral epithelium, which gives rise to further invagination of the vestibular and the dental lamina, has become clefted orally: the formation the oral vestibule has begun.

3.4.4 Primordium of m^1 (Figs 29 and 30)

The cap m^1 is the largest primordium of this fetus. The anterior part of the circular bulging of this cap is the most prominent and ascends in a cranial direction. In caudal and lateral directions it merges into the sturdy lateral enamel lamina. The entire cap is clearly tilted in a posterior and medial direction. As can be seen from the lateral aspect (Fig 29), another epithelial ledge runs between the lateral enamel lamina and the oral epithelium; thus a very deep enamel niche is formed. The posterior marginal bulge of the cap m^1 is thinner and does not ascend as high as the anterior bulge. The lateral margin ascends even less and a medial marginal bulge is not present, so the cap is open in the medial direction. The anterior enamel niche of this molar primordium is much deeper than the lateral enamel bulge. The reason is the mighty anterior marginal bulge, which rises so high and extends so far anteriorly. The enamel knot is just a flat, wide protrusion.
In the region between the canine and the molar primordia there is a voluminous extension of the maxilla reaching down approximately 20 μm to the vestibular lamina. A smaller, more laterally running extension lies at a distance of 150 μm from the mesial part of the cap m^1, while the distance in a cranial direction is about 200 μm. There is no bone distal to the primordium of m^1.

3.4.5 Primordium of m^2 (Figs 29 and 38)

The primordium of the second primary molar resembles the flat cap stage without a prominent enamel knot. The cap is tilted slightly in a medial direction. The anterior epithelial mass of the cap has formed a marginal bulge that runs obliquely in a medioposterior direction. It leans well above the

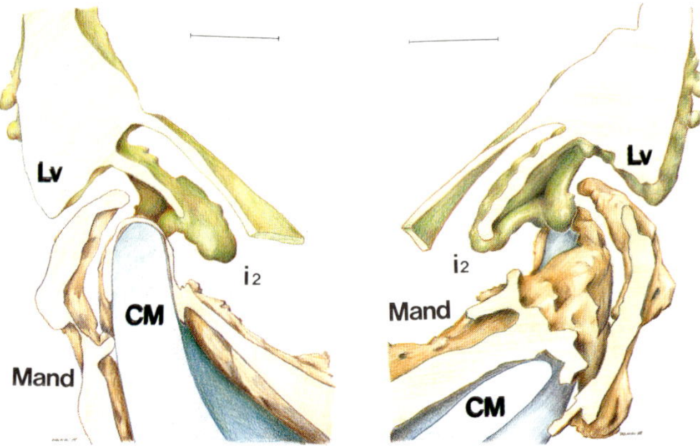

Fig 31 a The same fetus (47 mm). Partial reconstruction, shown in a medial view, illustrates the spatial relationship between the right cap i_2, the vestibular lamina (Lv), and the mandible (Mand), which almost completely covers Meckel's cartilage (CM). Scale: 250 μm.

Fig 31 b The same reconstruction, lateral view. Scale: 250 μm.

oral epithelium, forming a deep enamel trough medially. Toward the medial margin of the cap, the bulge clearly decreases in height and runs further distally. The bulge of the lateral part of the cap is almost evenly thick. The lateral enamel lamina is very short in this region because the entire cap does not protrude very far into the mesenchyme. There is a longer and more expanded epithelial ledge that runs from the posterior end of the cap in an oral and medial direction; thus, it forms the distal border of the enamel niche. The mesial enamel niche is larger and deeper than the lateral enamel niche.

Maxillary bone above the primordium of the second primary molar lies as far away as 500 μm.

3.4.6 Primordium of i_1 (Figs 30 and 39)

The primordium of the mandibular central primary incisor has reached the cap stage without a distinctly protruding enamel knot. The marginal bulge is well developed, but toward the distal side of the cap it levels out so that the trough of the cap has no distal wall. As seen from a caudal direction, the primordium has an oval shape, showing the greatest diameter mesiodistally. The lateral enamel lamina is bulky and thus forms a deep enamel niche distally inferior to the cap. At the mesial side of the primordium, there is a shallow enamel trough, as a consequence of the prominence of the mesial marginal bulge of the cap and oblique direction of the lateral enamel lamina. In the sulcus between the cap i_1 and the vestibular lamina is an additional ledge, obviously the *Nebenleiste* described by Bolk (1913). Its extension is limited only to the region of the primordium i_1.

The vestibular lamina extends below the primordium for about 50 μm. There are extensions of mandibular bone that protrude into the space between the vestibular lamina and the cap i_1. The distance to the vestibular lamina is about 70 μm, whereas to the tooth primordium it is not less than 125 μm. Whereas some extensions of the mandibular bone cover the anterior part of Meckel's cartilage, its surface facing the cap remains bone-free. Its distance to the cap i_1 is about 140 μm.

3.4.7 Primordium of i_2 (Figs 31 and 40)

As previously described, the position of the maxillary lateral incisor is farther away from the dental lamina than the central incisor. The same is true for the situation in the mandibular region, where the cap i_2 is located at a greater distance from the vestibular lamina than the cap i_1. The primordium i_2 has reached the cap stage without a protruding enamel knot. As seen from a caudal direction, this cap is not as oval as the cap i_1, but it is more rounded. The marginal bulge of the cap is well developed around the whole periphery of the cap, but in the distal part of the cap it is particularly thin, yet still visible. The lateral enamel lamina of Bolk (1913) is more bulky than that of i_1. It inserts further laterally at the cap and, corresponding to

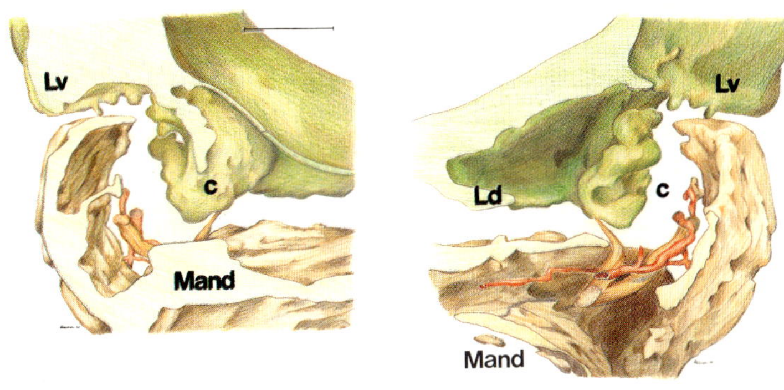

Fig 32a The same fetus (47 mm). Partial reconstuction, illustrates the spatial relationship between the right cap c_1, the vestibular lamina (Lv), the mandible (Mand), and nerves and vessels. Medial view. Scale: 250 μm.

Fig 32b Lateral view of the same reconstruction. Scale: 250 μm.

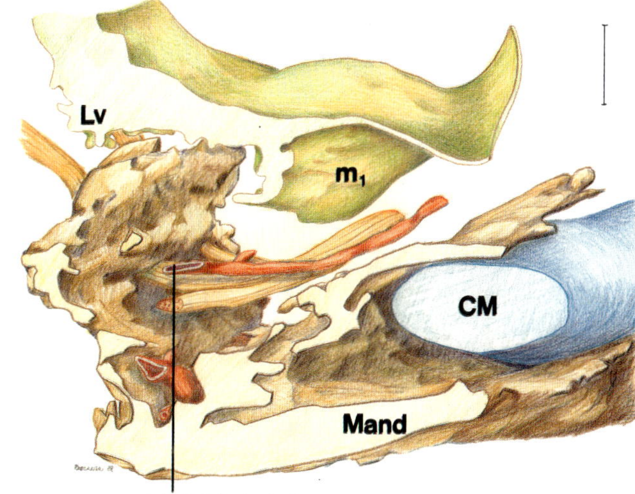

Fig 33a The same fetus (47 mm). Partial reconstruction illustrates the spatial relationship between the right cap m_1, the vestibular lamina (Lv), Meckel's cartilage (CM), the mandible (Mand), and nerves and vessels. Medial view. Scale: 250 μm.

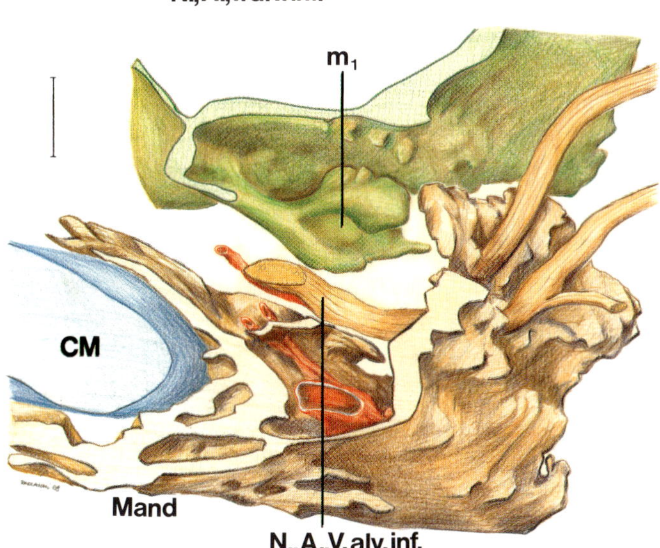

Fig 33b Lateral view of the same reconstruction. Scale: 250 μm.

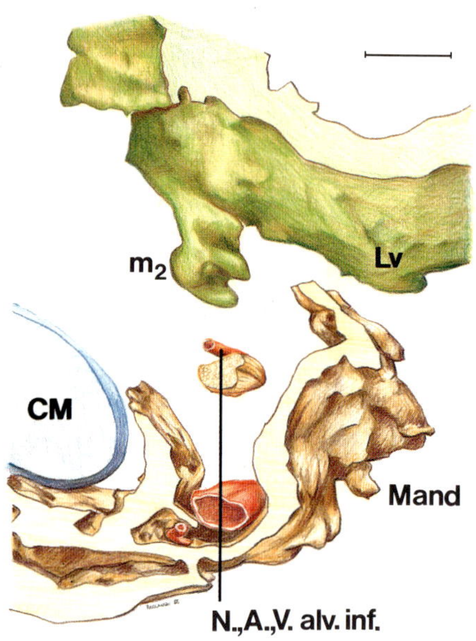

Fig 34 The same fetus (47 mm). Partial reconstruction illustrates the spatial relationship between the right cap m_2, the vestibular lamina (Lv), Meckel's cartilage (CM), the mandible (Mand), and the nerves (N, A, V alv inf). Medial view. Scale: 250 μm.

the greater distance, it extends further into the sulcus between the cap and the vestibular lamina. In this way a large, distally open and markedly confined enamel niche has been formed. As a consequence of the relatively large lateral enamel lamina, there is a clearly visible enamel trough at the mesial side of the cap i_2. The primordium of i_2 extends deeper than the vestibular lamina for about 100 to 200 μm.

The most anterior and cranial part of the mandibular bone of this region projects deeply into the sulcus between the vestibular lamina and the primordium i_2. It maintains a distance of only about 50 μm to the epithelium.

The mandibular bone is not completely continuous in this region because a deep and narrow gap has formed between that part of the mandibular bone just described and the portion that covers Meckel's cartilage. As soon as the anterior part of Meckel's cartilage descends caudally, this gap becomes wider to form a groove in a lateral direction.

Whereas Meckel's cartilage is as well developed because it is below the cap i_1 in the mesial region beneath i_2, it is covered by a layer of bone, which is 15 to 100 μm thick toward the distal part of the primordial region. Here the distance to i_2 is about 130 μm.

3.4.8 Primordium of c_1 (Figs 32 and 41)

The primordium of the mandibular primary canine has reached the cap stage, with a well-shaped enamel knot and a voluminous marginal bulge. Distally the cap is open, because there the marginal bulge is very thin and barely protrudes. The outline of the cap is triangular, with one tip pointing mesially and the longest margin running parallel to the vestibular lamina. The lateral enamel lamina is well developed and contributes to the formation of a deep enamel niche. The entire cap is bent anteriorly and laterally. When seen from the mesial aspect, the enamel trough is only weakly developed. In this region, the cap c_1 extends lower than the vestibular lamina for about 300 μm.

The cleft of the mandible, which has been described as commencing as a narrow gap caudal to the primordium i_2, is continuous laterally and becomes a wide bony groove in this region. The cap c_1 descends into this groove. The distance between the primordium and the bone in a vestibular direction is about 270 μm; in a caudal direction, it is about 120 μm. In the depth of the bony groove run anterior branches of the inferior alveolar nerves and blood vessels.

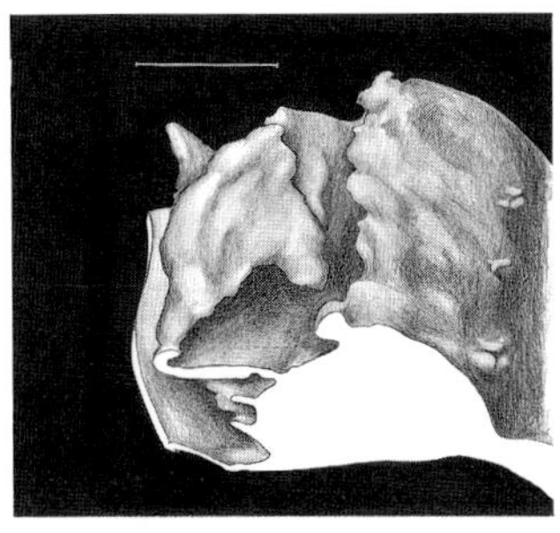

Fig 35 Embryo, 47 mm. Reconstruction of the right primordium i^1, lateral and 60° cranial view. In the right half of the figure runs the vestibular lamina, and at its right margin there are additional invaginations of the epithelium, which represent the early primordia of the labial glands. Scale: 250 μm.

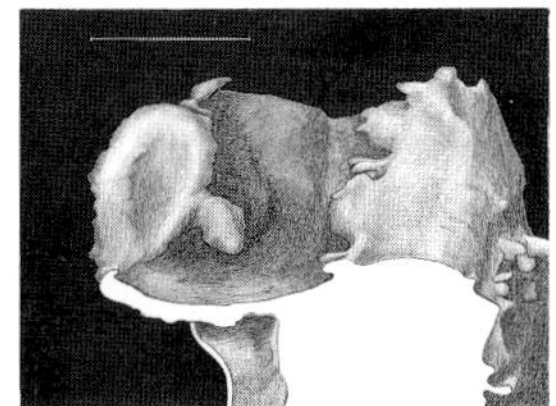

Fig 36 The same fetus (47 mm). Reconstruction of the right primordium i^2. Lateral and 60° cranial view. Scale: 250 μm.

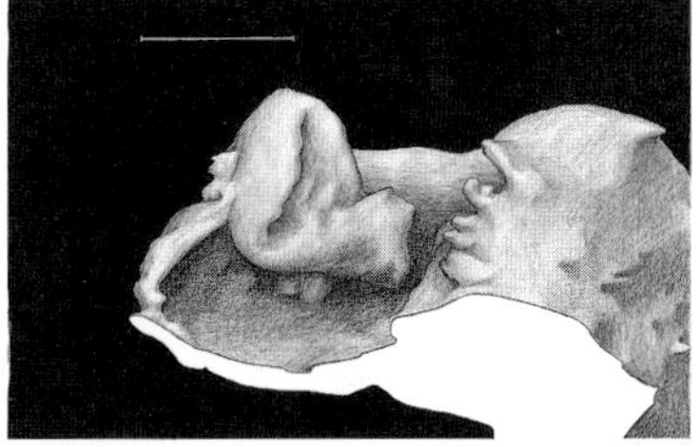

Fig 37 The same fetus (47 mm). Reconstruction of the right primordium c^1. Lateral and 60° cranial view. Scale: 250 μm.

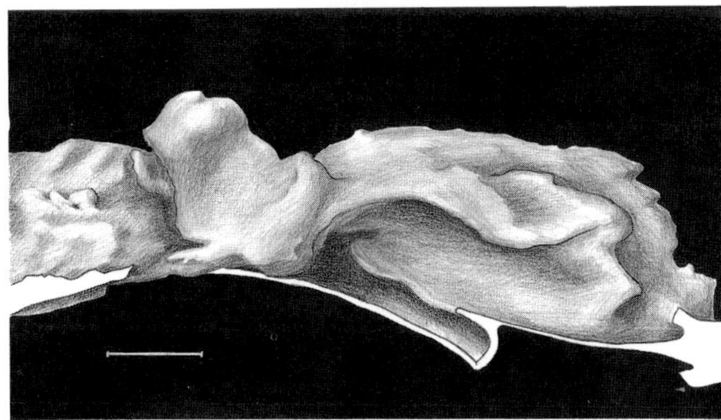

Fig 38 The same fetus (47 mm). Reconstruction of the right primordia m^1 (left) and m^2 (right). Medial and 45° cranial view. Scale: 250 μm.

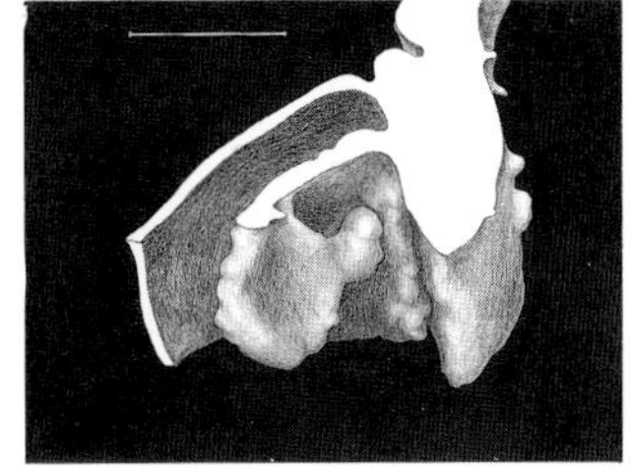

Fig 39 The same fetus (47 mm). Reconstruction of the right primordium i_1. Lateral and 45° caudal view. Scale: 250 μm.

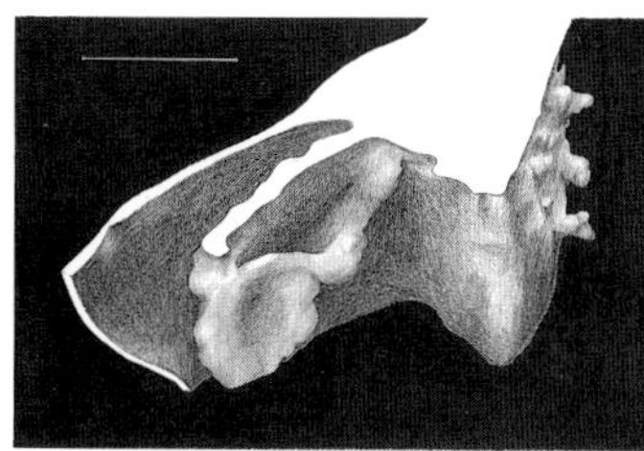

Fig 40 The same fetus (47 mm). Reconstruction of the right primordium i_2. Lateral and 45° caudal view. Scale: 250 μm.

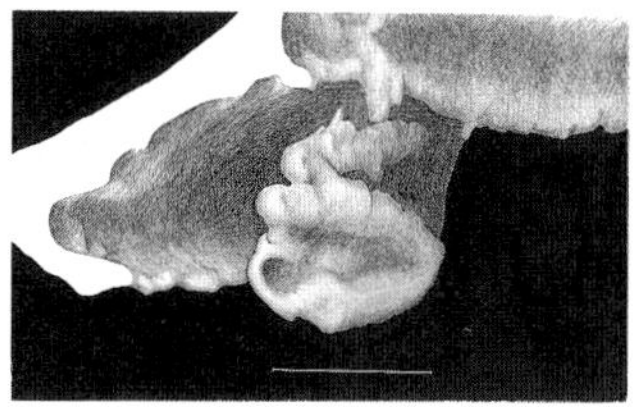

Fig 41 The same fetus (47 mm). Reconstruction of the right primordium c_1. Lateral and 45° caudal view. Scale: 250 μm.

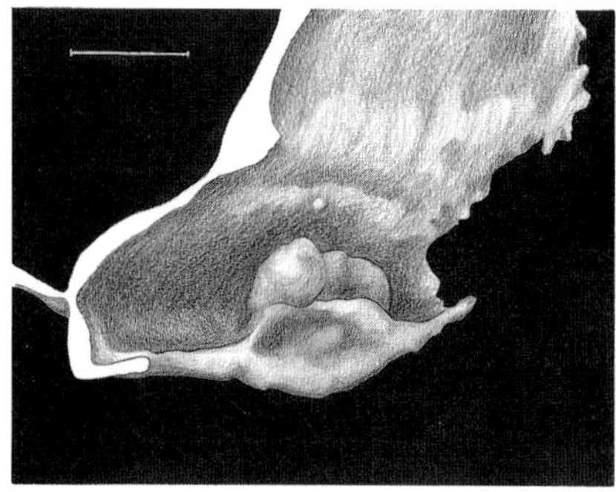

Fig 42 The same fetus (47 mm). Reconstruction of the right primordium m_1. Lateral, 30° anterior, and 45° caudal view. Scale: 250 μm.

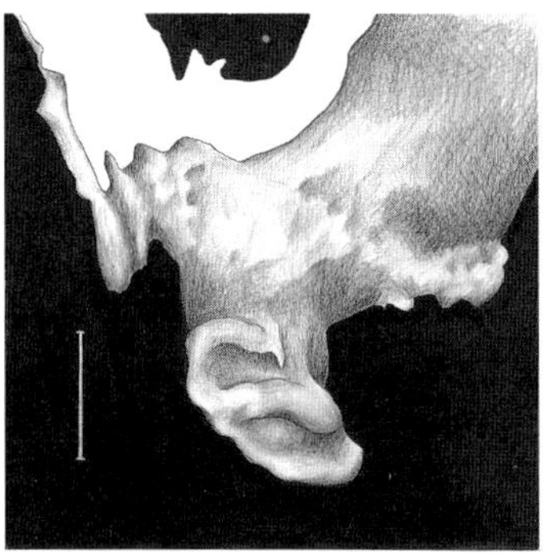

Fig 43 The same fetus (47 mm). Reconstruction of the right primordium m_2. Lateral, 60° anterior, and 30° caudal view. Scale: 250 μm.

3.4.9 Primordium of m_1 (Figs 33 and 42)

The primordium of the mandibular first primary molar has reached the cap stage. It can be compared to the outline of a flattened pentagon, which extends more in a mesiodistal direction. Two tips are close to the bulky lateral enamel lamina, two further tips merge mesially and distally into the general dental lamina, and a fifth tip, just visible, is located almost in the center of the medial margin of the cap m_1 (Fig 42). The enamel knot is clearly protruded, and the whole primordium is tilted in a lateral direction. The marginal bulge follows the outline of the cap without interruptions, but its thickness varies: the medial bulge is almost as thick as the general dental lamina and, because the cap is tilted, protrudes farthest into the mesenchyme. At the mesial side of the cap m_1 the marginal bulge maintains its thickness, but running to the lateral margin of the cap it becomes thinner. In this same region, the lateral enamel lamina is voluminous and bulky and protrudes over the brim of the cap. It runs obliquely between the cap and the oral epithelium, with its distal part lying closer to the cap. Thus, distally as well as mesially, a deep enamel niche is formed. In this region the vestibular lamina is not invaginated very deeply.

The mandibular groove, into which the primordium m_1 descends, is about 750 μm wide and almost 1 mm deep. The lateral part of the mandible runs caudally beneath the vestibular lamina and comes up as close as about 175 μm to m_1. The bone lying medial to the bony groove covers Meckel's cartilage, but toward the oral cavity Meckel's cartilage is free of bone. Laterally and medially, the distance between the bone and the primordium is about 250 μm. Caudally the distance to the deepest spot of the bony groove is about 800 μm. The inferior alveolar nerve runs in the mandibular groove, exiting through the mental foramen laterally. In addition, several inferior alveolar arteries run in the groove, and the homonymous vein extends along the bottom of the groove.

3.4.10 Primordium of m_2 (Figs 34 and 43)

The cap of the mandibular second primary molar is characterized by a well-developed enamel knot and voluminous marginal bulges, but its overall size is smaller than that of m_1, just described. In addition, the form of the two molar primordia is different: the cap m_2 shows more the outline of a rhomb. The lateral enamel lamina merges directly into the circular bulge at the distal end of the primordium. The lateral enamel lamina then describes a curve, first in a cranial and then in an anterior direction. At the same time it marks the distal end of the dental lamina. The enamel niche is relatively shallow and small at the mesial aspect of the primordium; distally there is no enamel niche, because here the bulges and ledges are too flat. Whereas in the primordium of m_1 the *lateral* part of the marginal bulge was the thinnest, it is the distal and *medial* portion that is the thinnest in the primordium of m_2. It is, however, high enough to fence the cap distally. Conversely, in an anterior direction, the trough of cap m_2 is open, because here the bulge is locally very flat. The whole primordium m_2 is tilted in a lateral direction. In a distance of 600 μm further laterally there are some single epithelial bulges that indicate the position of a vestibular lamina. Distally from the primordium, a much more distinct epithelial invagination (Fig 34, upper left corner) can be seen, which, because of its position, may not be the vestibular lamina.

Beneath the primordium of the second primary molar, the mandible forms a groove, similar to the situation around the primordium of m_1. The bony groove is continuous, so there is no bone between the two molar primordia; thus, in this fetus, none of the primordia is encased by bony partitions. The lateral edge of the mandible comes as close as 150 μm to the epithelial formations of the vestibular lamina. The distance between the molar primordium and the deepest part of the bony groove is slightly more than 1 mm. The medial edge of the mandibular groove covers the lateral aspect of Meckel's cartilage, but is not as wide as underneath the primordium of m_1. Therefore, Meckel's cartilage faces the primordium of m_2 with one surface lying at a distance of about 470 μm.

3.5 Early bell stage

The description of this stage refers to the reconstruction of the fetus VER (64 mm CRL), in which most of the primordia are in the early bell stage.

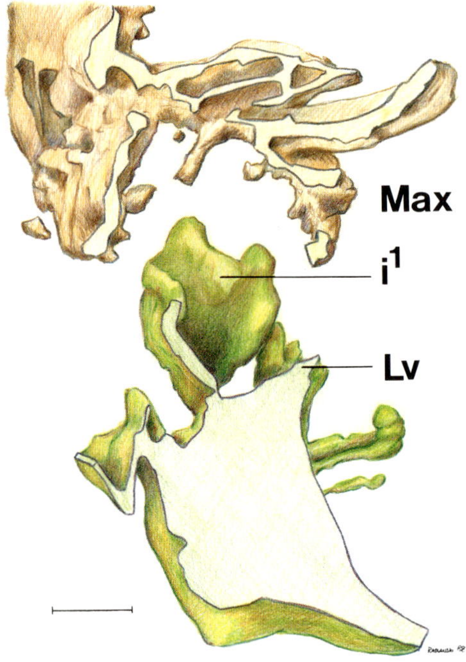

Fig 44 Embryo, 64 mm. Partial reconstruction illustrates the spatial relationship between the right bell i^1, the vestibular lamina (Lv), and the maxilla (Max). Lateral view. Scale: 250 μm.

3.5.1 Primordium of i^1 (Figs 44, 53, and 62)

The primordium of i^1 has reached the stage of the early bell in the fetus of 64 mm CRL. It rises above the vestibular lamina for about two thirds of its size, and it projects markedly anteriorly and distally. As in the earlier stages, where the distance of i^1 to the vestibular lamina is always smaller than the distance between i^2 and the vestibular lamina, the distance is also particularly small in the early bell stage. The primordium is flattened along the dental arch, its mesiodistal diameter being clearly greater than its vestibulo-oral one. The lateral enamel lamina arises from the rim of the bell, slightly more distally, before it turns mesially and inserts into the general dental lamina. Thus, a funnel-shaped deep enamel niche is formed distally, and mesially there is a shallow enamel trough.

A sagittal section (Figs 62a and b) shows the contour of the bell's epithelium facing the early mesenchymal papilla. (Later these cells become the ameloblasts of the inner enamel epithelium and secrete the enamel matrix.) The epithelium of the bell is invaginated from a cranial direction almost to the middle of the primordium. At its deepest point the epithelial contour describes a comparatively sharp curve. From this point in a palatal direction, the contour describes an obvious inflection, which seems to resemble the palatal concavity of the completed tooth.

The epithelial excrescences that arise from the labial aspect of the vestibular lamina are the primordia of the labial glands. In this stage they clearly resemble the ducts and the endpieces (Fig 53).

The mesenchyme surrounding the primordium is greatly condensed. Around this condensed mesenchyme, which will give rise to the early dental papilla, the maxillary bone forms a corresponding cavity. The distance between bone and the primordium of i^1 in a cranial direction is about 300 μm, and in a labial and palatal direction, it is about 160 μm.

3.5.2 Primordium of i^2 (Figs 45, 54, and 63)

The primordium of the maxillary lateral primary incisor is clearly smaller and less developed when

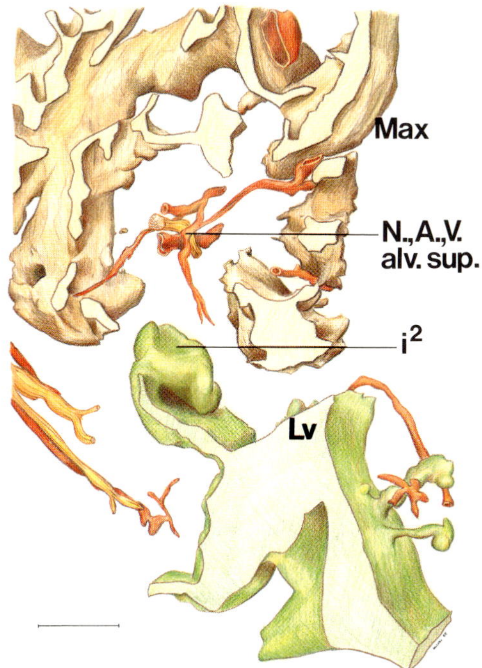

Fig 45 The same fetus (64 mm). Partial reconstruction illustrates the spatial relationship between the right cap i^2, the vestibular lamina (Lv), the maxilla (Max), and nerves and vessels (N, A, V alv sup). Lateral view. Scale: 250 μm.

compared to the primordium of i^1, just described. It may be staged as a late cap. Like the other incisor primordia, it is inclined anteriorly and distally. Its distance from the vestibular lamina is greater than that of i^1. The primordium i^2 rises almost completely above the vestibular lamina. The form of the tooth bell is only slightly oval, since the vestibulo-oral diameter is 220 μm, and the mesiodistal diameter is 290 μm. In this primordium, the lateral enamel lamina (Bolk 1913) inserts somewhat further distally (Fig 54) than in the primordium of i^1; thus, a marked enamel niche is formed distally, whereas mesially there is only a shallow trough. The vestibular lamina is cleft deeply from the oral direction in this region. Toward the middle of the primordium the cleft reaches almost down to the bottom of the epithelial invagination (Fig 63).

In sagittal section the contour of the future inner enamel epithelium shows a shallow concavity in sagittal section, which is typical for the cap stage without an enamel knot (Fig 63).

The bony cavity cranial to the primordium i^2 has a vertical diameter of about 1,000 μm, so it is greater in cranial direction than that of primordium i^1. The distance between the primordium and the bone in a palatal direction is about 130 μm, and in a vestibular direction it is 160 μm. Anterior extensions of maxillary bone extend down into the epithelial sulcus between primordium and vestibular lamina, coming as close as 150 μm.

3.5.3 Primordium of c^1 (Figs 46, 55, and 64)

The maxillary canine primordium of this fetus has reached the early bell stage and is well inclined in an anterior and distal direction. It rises completely above the vestibular lamina. There are some places where the epithelium of the bell is already separated from the general dental lamina. The rim of the bell is very low distally. The lateral enamel lamina arises directly anterior to this distal area and extends medially. Thus, the enamel niche beneath the tooth bell is very large and deep. The epithelial protrusion at the transition from the rim to the lateral enamel lamina is very prominent, and so there

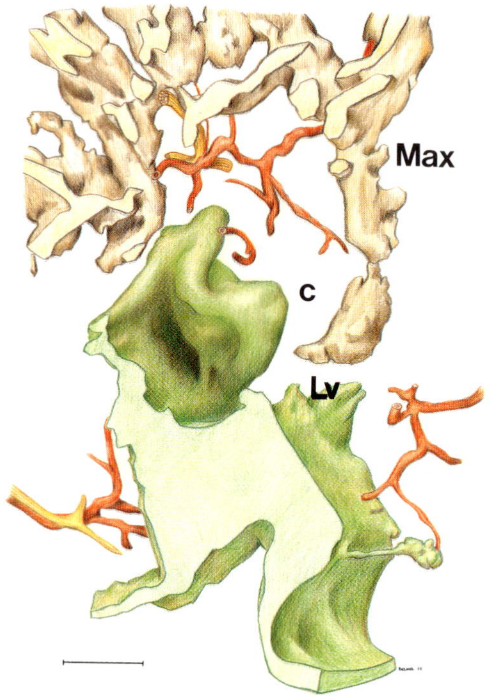

Fig 46 The same fetus (64 mm). Partial reconstruction illustrates the spatial relationship between the right bell c^1, the vestibular lamina (Lv), the maxilla (Max), and nerves and vessels. Lateral view. Scale: 250 μm.

results a triangular outline for the cavity of the tooth bell (Fig 55). One apex of the triangle points distally.

What will eventually be the inner enamel epithelium of this canine tooth bell has a concavity at the palatal contour of the epithelium that can be seen in sagittal section (Fig 64). It is slightly deeper than that of i^1.

In the region of the canine primordium, there is a distance of only 90 μm between the anterior extension of the maxilla and the vestibular lamina, much less than found in the region anterior to i^2. The distance between the palatal extensions of maxillary bone and the canine primordium is about 190 μm, in the cranial direction the distance is 530 μm. The reconstruction in Fig 46 shows that the canine primordium is more enclosed by bone than are the two incisor primordia. At the margins of the protrusions of maxillary bone, areas with increased numbers of osteoclasts could be observed.

3.5.4 Primordium of m^1 (Figs 47, 56, and 65)

The first maxillary molar has reached the early bell stage. The primordium is strongly inclined in a distal direction and extends completely above the vestibular lamina. As a consequence of the arrangement of the lateral enamel lamina, mesially there is a deep enamel niche (Figs 47 and 56), and distally there is only a shallow trough beneath the primordium. The tooth bell has an almost square outline, and at the medial and distal margin of the rim there are two distinct bulging epithelial formations, of which the lateral is higher than the medial (Figs 56 and 65). The contour of the epithelium at the inside of the bell shows a curvature in which the vertex is not located in the middle of the bell, but more toward the anterior part. It is thus positioned just above the attachment of the tooth bell to the general dental lamina. In this way the whole primordium appears to be extended more posteriorly than anteriorly.

Between the maxillary canine primordium and the primordium m^1, a large extension of the maxilla

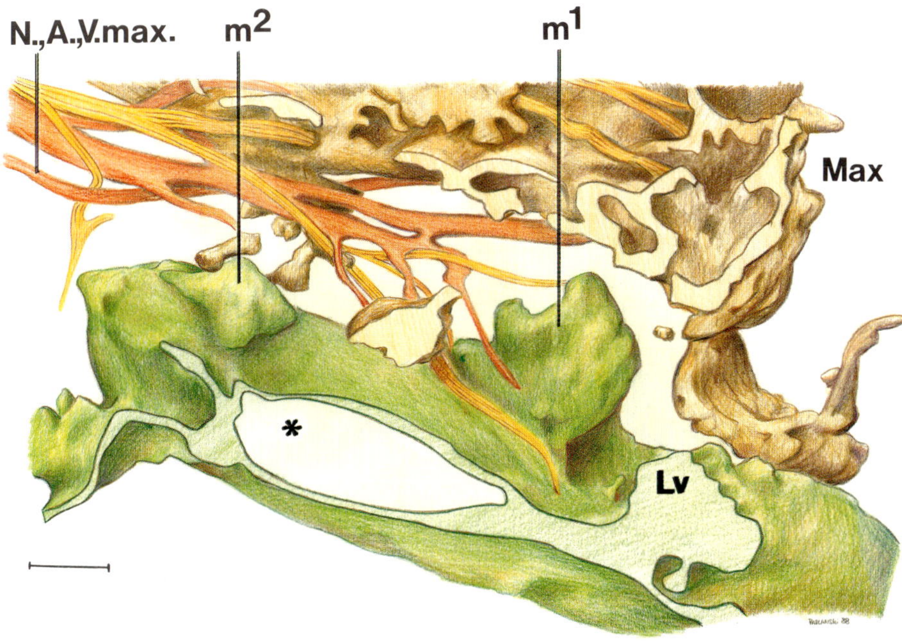

Fig 47 The same fetus (64 mm). Partial reconstruction illustrates the spatial relationship between the right bell m^1 and the cap m^2, the vestibular lamina (Lv), the maxilla (Max), and the nerves and vessels (N, A, V max). Lateral view. Asterisk denotes cut surface of the mesenchyme cranial to the oral cavity. This cut surface is due to the wide medial extension of the dental epithelium. Scale: 250 μm.

descends toward the vestibular lamina as close as 140 μm. The depth of the maxillary bony cavity above the primordium m^1 ranges between 380 and 540 μm. In addition, there are bony formations located between the two molar primordia m^1 and m^2. The distance between the bone and the bell m^1 is about 500 μm; the distance from the bone to the oral epithelium is about 195 μm.

3.5.5 Primordium of m^2 (Figs 47, 56, and 66)

This primordium has not yet attained the early bell stage. A late cap best describes the primordium of the maxillary second primary molar. An enamel knot is just visible. The complete primordium is inclined more medially than distally. Because the lateral enamel lamina is located almost in the middle of the primordium, an enamel niche has form ed from the mesial as well as from the distal aspects. In a cranial direction, the lateral enamel lamina merges into the bulging brim of the cap, which here is thickened cranially. The outline of the cap almost resembles a trapezoid, of which the longest edge lies laterally, and the shortest medially. In a sagittal section, the inner contour of the cap represents a shallow trough, which is characterized by wavy indentations on its posterior aspect. Distal to the cap the dental lamina continues for about half the distance of the cap's diameter, before bending sharply in a caudal direction.

The body of the maxillary bone is located at about 540 μm cranial to the primordium, although some single bony formations are found closer to the primordium in mesial and lateral directions (Fig 47).

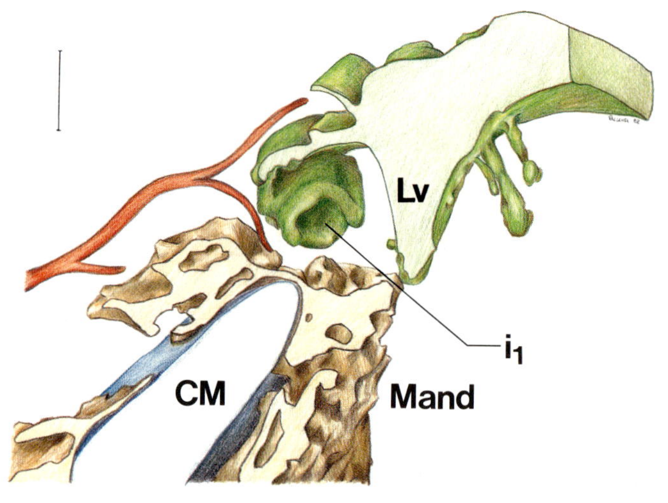

Fig 48 The same fetus (64 mm). Partial reconstruction illustrates the spatial relationship between the right bell i_1, the vestibular lamina (Lv), the mandible (Mand), Meckel's cartilage (CM), and some vessels. Lateral view. Scale: 250 μm.

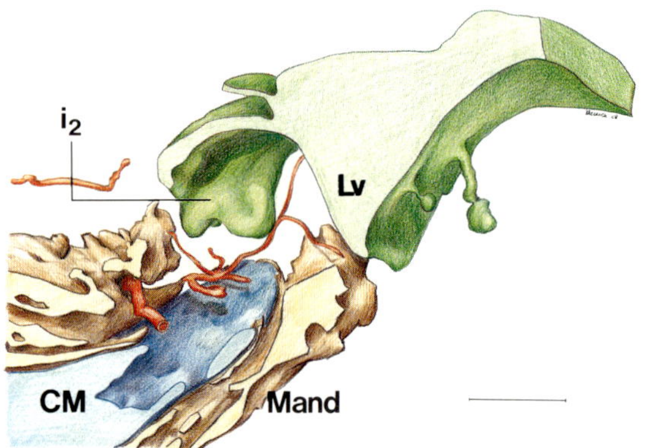

Fig 49 The same fetus (64 mm). Partial reconstruction illustrates the spatial relationship between the right bell i_2, the vestibular lamina (Lv), the mandible (Mand), Meckel's cartilage (CM), and some vessels. Lateral view. Scale: 250 μm.

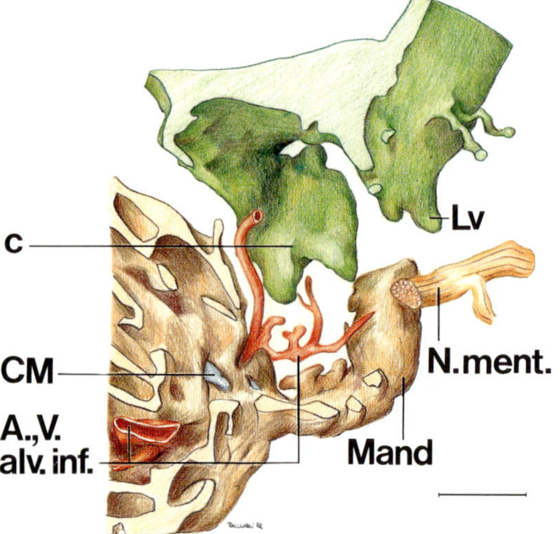

Fig 50 The same fetus (64 mm). Partial reconstruction illustrates the spatial relationship between the right bell c_1, the vestibular lamina (Lv), the mandible (Mand), vessels and nerves (A, V alv inf, N ment), and Meckel's cartilage (CM). Lateral view. Scale: 250 μm.

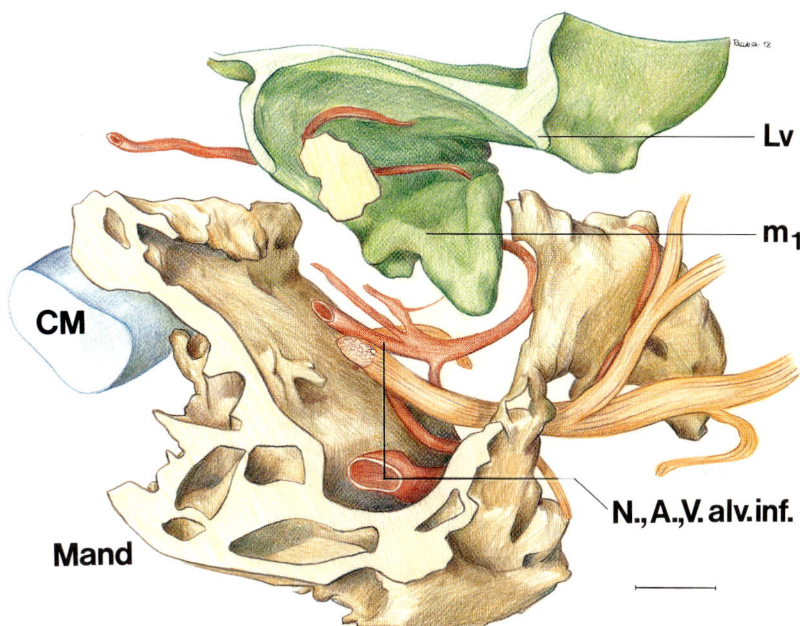

Fig 51 The same fetus (64 mm). Partial reconstruction illustrates the spatial relationship between the right bell m_1, the vestibular lamina (Lv), the mandible (Mand), vessels and nerves (A, V alv inf), and Meckel's cartilage (CM). Lateral view. Scale: 250 μm.

3.5.6 Primordium of i_1 (Figs 48, 57, and 67)

In this fetus the primordium of the primary mandibular central incisor has reached the bell stage. It is inclined distally and here forms a deep enamel niche beneath the primordium. In this region the vestibular lamina is invaginated so far into the mesenchyme that it extends beyond the primordium for about one third of its invaginational depth. This primordium is much wider mesiodistally than vestibulo-orally, so it is clearly oval. The contour of the inner enamel epithelium of the tooth bell shows (more markedly than with the primordium i^1) a clear indentation on its lingual convexity.

Directly caudal to the primordium, at a distance of about 130 μm, lies Meckel's cartilage. It is covered locally by a thin layer of mandibular bone, whereas underneath the primordium of i_1 there remain some areas free of bone.

At its lingual, as well as at its vestibular sides, Meckel's cartilage is covered by bulky masses of mandibular bone, which approach the primordium as close as 85 μm from the lingual side and 65 μm from the vestibular side.

3.5.7 Primordium of i_2 (Figs 49, 58, and 68)

The primordium of the primary second mandibular incisor has reached the early bell stage. It is not inclined distally like most of the other primordia of this fetus, but its distal rim is slightly retracted. Between the primordium and the general dental lamina, the lateral enamel lamina is spread out and contributes distally to the formation of a deep enamel niche. This lateral enamel lamina projects further distally at i_2 than at i_1.

The outline of the bell is only slightly oval mesiodistally when viewed from below: the mesiodistal diameter of 280 μm contrasts with a vestibulo-oral diameter of only 240 μm. In sagittal section, the contour shows a regular invagination of that part of the epithelium that faces the mesenchymal papilla.

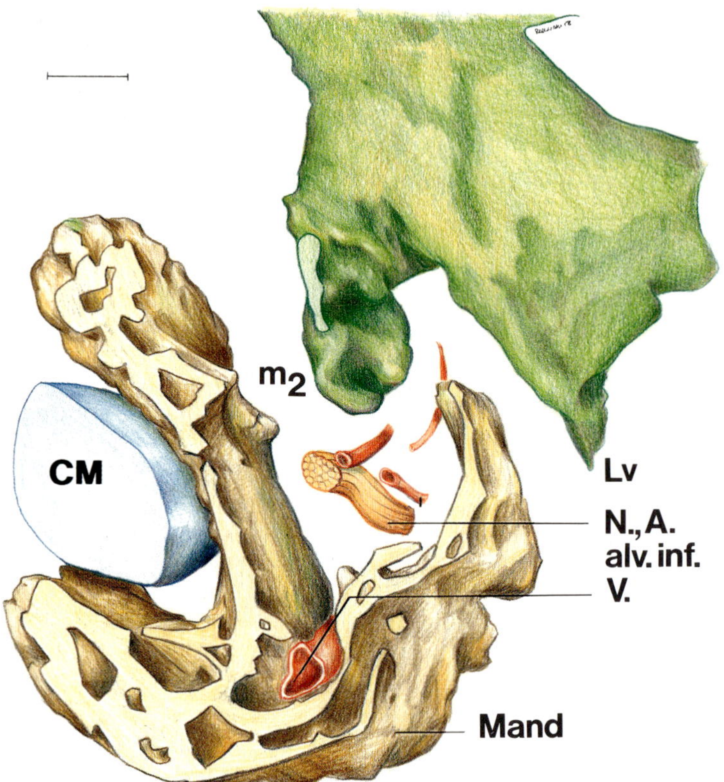

Fig 52 The same fetus (64 mm). Partial reconstruction illustrates the spatial relationship between the right bell m_2, the vestibular lamina (Lv), the mandible (Mand), vessels and nerves (A, V alv inf), and Meckel's cartilage (CM). Lateral view. Scale: 250 μm.

Inferior to the primordium, Meckel's cartilage already reveals signs of resorption and looks excavated. In the middle area of the primordium the distance between the primordium and Meckel's cartilage is about 360 μm, and it increases in a distal direction. Mandibular bone comes closer to the tooth bell: lingually the distance is about 110 μm, and vestibularly it is about 120 μm.

3.5.8 Primordium of c_1 (Figs 50, 59, and 69)

In contrast to the incisor primordia nearly half of the canine's primordium can be found beyond the vestibular lamina. This primordium has reached the bell stage and its cellular connection to the general dental lamina is reduced to not more than four cells at some spots. The tooth bell is not inclined very far distally, but its distal rim is clearly retracted. The lateral enamel lamina forms a distal enamel niche, which is wider anteriorly than the corresponding enamel niche of the primordia i_2 and i_1. When viewed from below, the outline of this tooth bell is almost round, with some irregularities that result from the varying thicknes of the circular bulge. The sagittal section of this primordium reveals an even contour of the future inner enamel epithelium, with the sharpest curve being found at the deepest point of the concavity. Within the epithelium of the tooth bell next to a dispersion of the epithelium there can be found a cellular condensation that constitutes an enamel chord (*Schmelzstrang*, Ahrens 1913a).
In the region of the canine primordium, Meckel's cartilage is almost completely covered by mandibular bone, with only some solitary fenestrations remaining open. Laterally the mandible has formed a bony groove, containing the primordium of

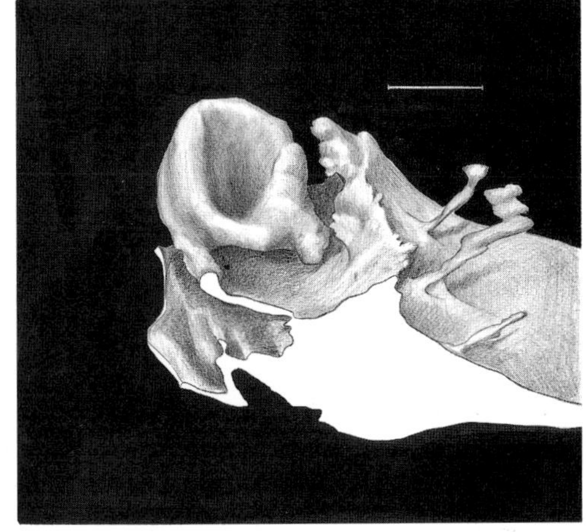

Fig 53 The same fetus (64 mm). Partial reconstruction of the primordium i^1, lateral and 60° cranial view. In the right half of the figure there runs the vestibular lamina, and at the right margin there arise early formations of labial glands. Scale: 250 μm.

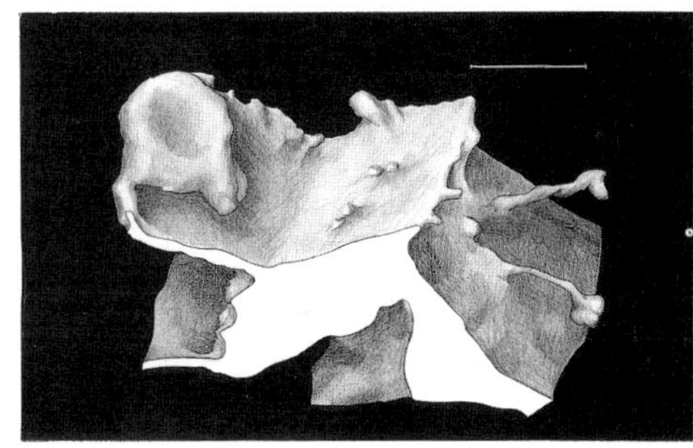

Fig 54 The same fetus (64 mm). Partial reconstruction of the primordium i^2. Lateral and 60° cranial view. Scale: 250 μm.

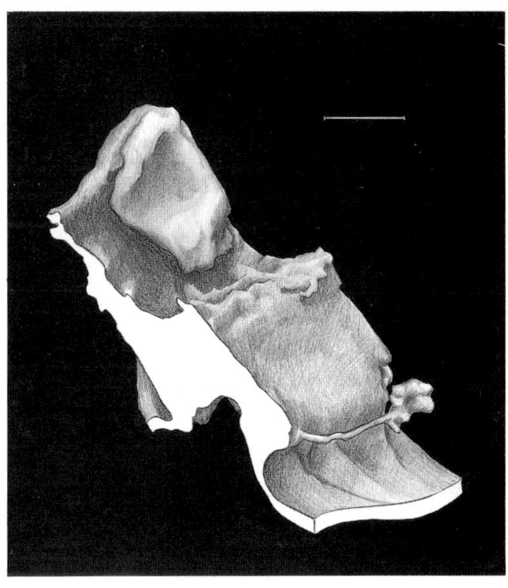

Fig 55 The same fetus (64 mm). Partial reconstruction of the primordium c^1. Lateral, 60° cranial, and 45° anterior view. Scale: 250 μm.

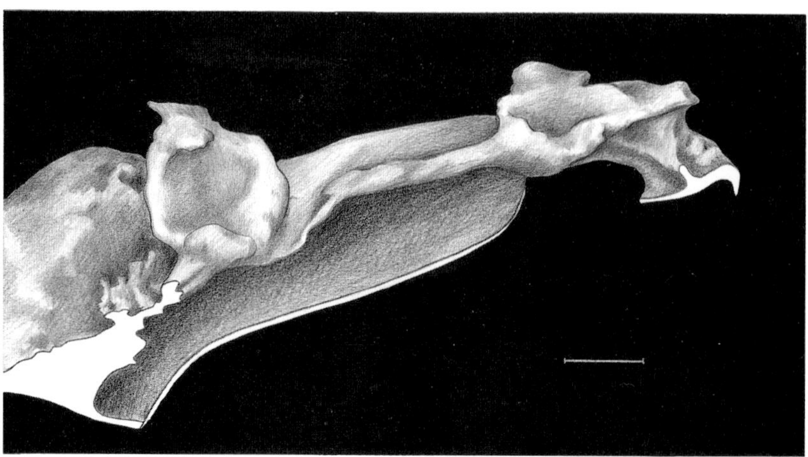

Fig 56 The same fetus (64 mm). Partial reconstruction of the primordium m^1 (left) and m^2 (right). Medial and 60° cranial view. Scale: 250 μm.

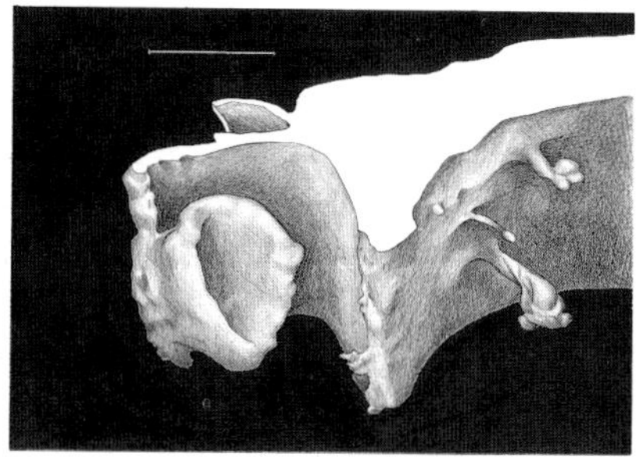

Fig 57 The same fetus (64 mm). Partial reconstruction of the primordium i_1. Lateral and 60° caudal view. Scale: 250 μm.

c_1. The distance to the floor of the groove is approximately 430 μm. The distance to the lingual wall is about 120 μm, and in the vestibular direction it is about 240 μm. The distance between the vestibular lamina and the lateral part of the bony groove is also about 240 μm.

3.5.9 Primordium of m_1 (Figs 51, 60, and 70)

The primordium of the mandibular first primary molar has reached the bell stage. It is slightly inclined posteriorly, and its bulging, anterior margin extends relatively far caudally. The lateral enamel lamina spreads out between this descending margin and the general dental lamina, thus forming an enamel niche. The posterior margin of the primordium is bulged, too, but it does not extend as far into the depth. The least protrusion is shown by the lateral rim of the primordium. In this region the vestibular lamina invaginates as a separate formation about 600 μm further laterally.

Between the anterior and the posterior rims the future inner enamel epithelium has an almost rectangular outline (Fig 60). In sagittal section, approximately through the middle of the primordium, it can be seen that the contour of the epithelium turns almost at a right angle; the epithelium between these two edges is curved slightly caudally, so there are formed two concavities and one convexity (Fig 70a).

The whole primordium m_1 lies in the bony groove

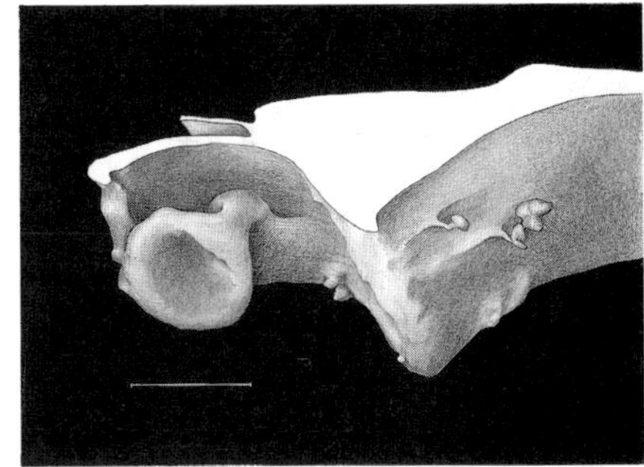

Fig 58 The same fetus (64 mm). Partial reconstruction of the primordium i_2. Lateral and 60° caudal view. Scale: 250 μm.

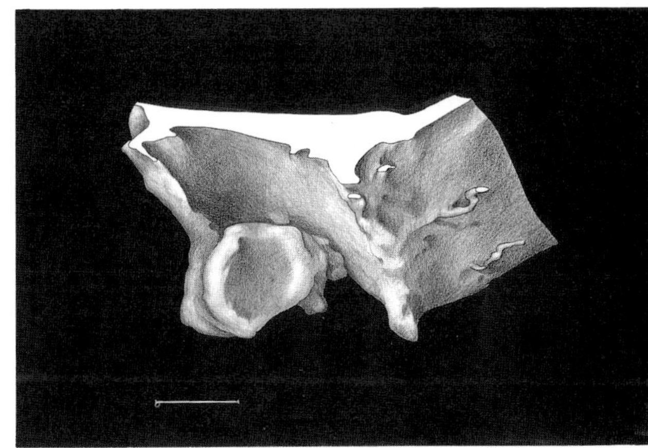

Fig 59 The same fetus (64 mm). Partial reconstruction of the primordium c_1. Lateral, 60° caudal, and 15° anterior view. Scale: 250 μm.

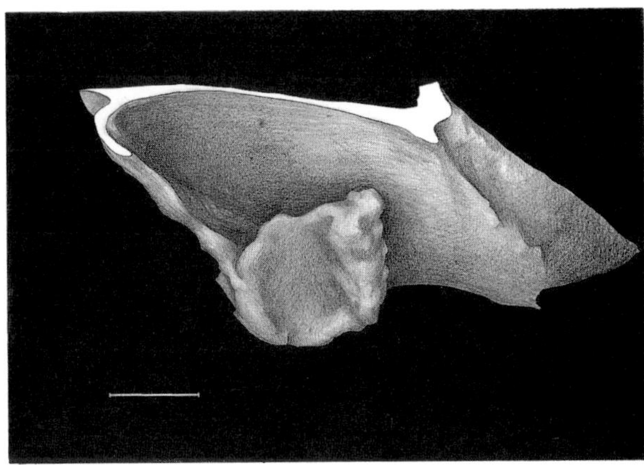

Fig 60 The same fetus (64 mm). Partial reconstruction of the primordium m_1. Lateral and 60° caudal view. Scale: 250 μm.

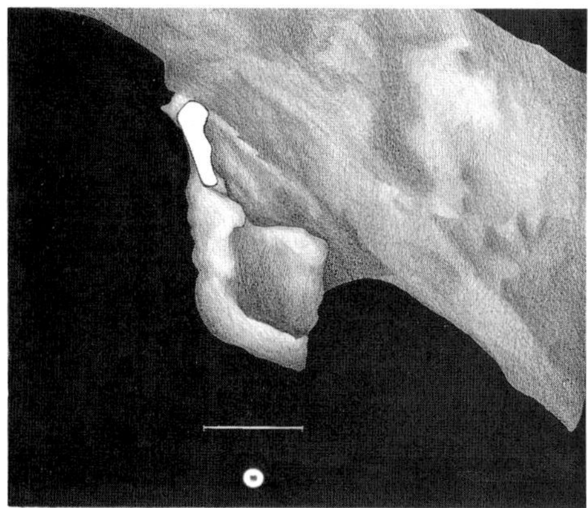

Fig 61 The same fetus (64 mm). Partial reconstruction of the primordium m_2. Lateral and 50° caudal view. Scale: 250 μm.

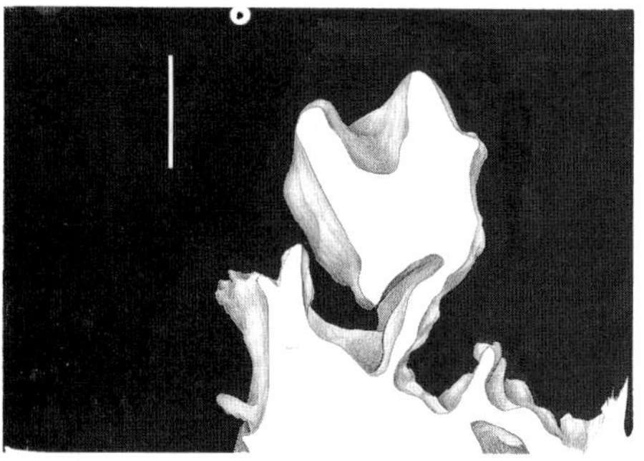

Fig 62a The same fetus (64 mm). Sagittally sectioned right primordium i^1. Right half, medial view. Scale: 250 μm.

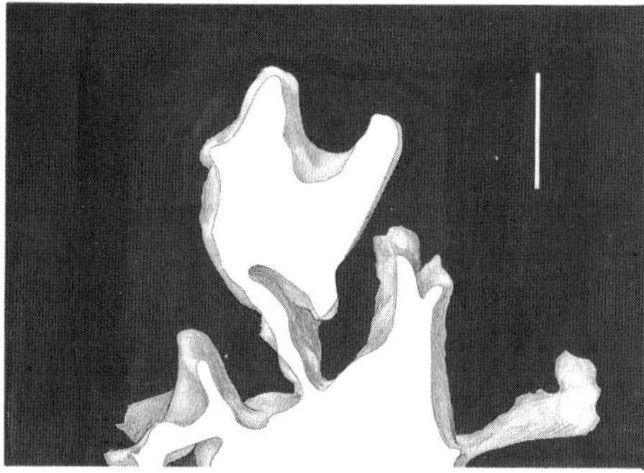

Fig 62b Left half of same primordium, lateral view. Scale: 250 μm.

of the mandible, descending for slightly more than half its length. The mandibular groove runs laterally from Meckel's cartilage and in this region has a maximum width of about 1,030 μm. The floor of the groove is approximately 870 μm away from the primordium, the distance to the anterior bony extension is about 100 μm, and the posterior distance is about 330 μm. Laterally, close to the position of the lateral enamel lamina, bone has formed at a distance of about 140 μm. The distance between the vestibular lamina and the lateral edge of the bony groove's confinement is about 170 μm. At the bottom of the bony groove the inferior alveolar vein is found. The homonymous nerve and artery course slightly above the floor (Fig 51).

3.5.10 Primordium of m_2 (Figs 52, 61, and 71)

The primordium of m_2 has reached the early bell stage, and it is relatively smaller than that of m_1. In contrast to the primordium of m_1, the primordium of m_2 inclines laterally and is open distally. Its outline is longish in a mesiodistal direction. Two laminae have formed between the primordium and the vestibular lamina.

One that runs closer to the tooth bell represents the lateral enamel lamina described by Bolk. Laterally, the enamel niche is formed between this lamina and the primordium. The other lamina runs above these epithelial structures and may be Bolk's (1913) *Nebenleiste*, which is seen only occasionally.

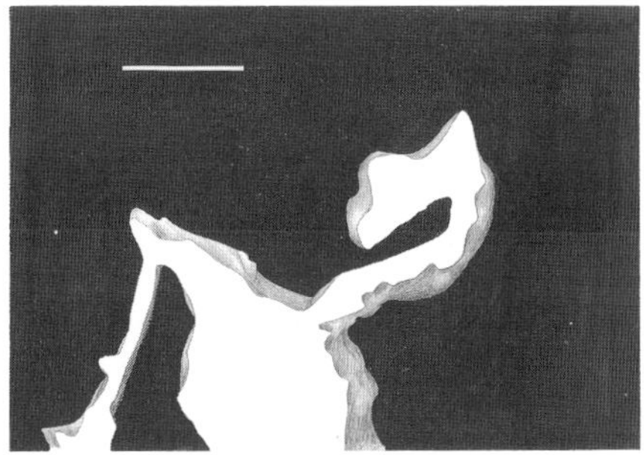

Fig 63a The same fetus (64 mm). Sagittally sectioned right primordium i^2. Right half, medial view. Scale: 250 μm.

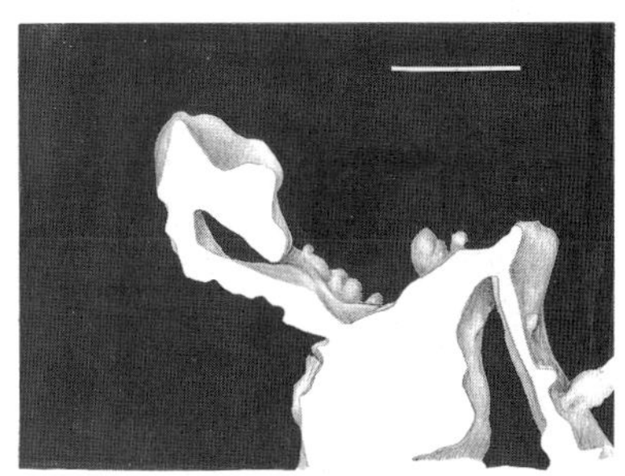

Fig 63b Left half of same primordium, lateral view. Scale: 250 μm.

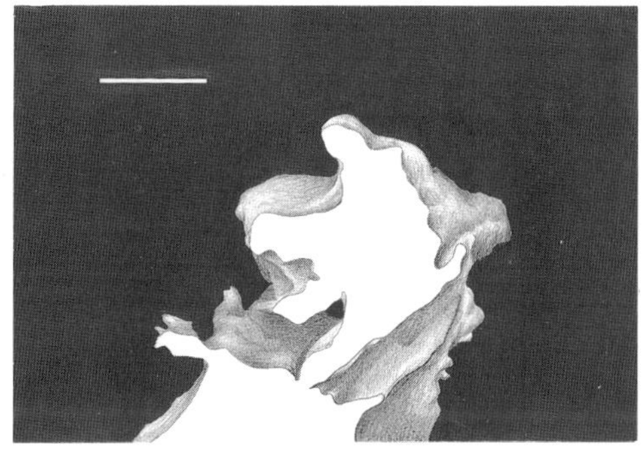

Fig 64a The same fetus (64 mm). Sagittally sectioned right primordium c^1. Right half, medial view. Scale: 250 μm.

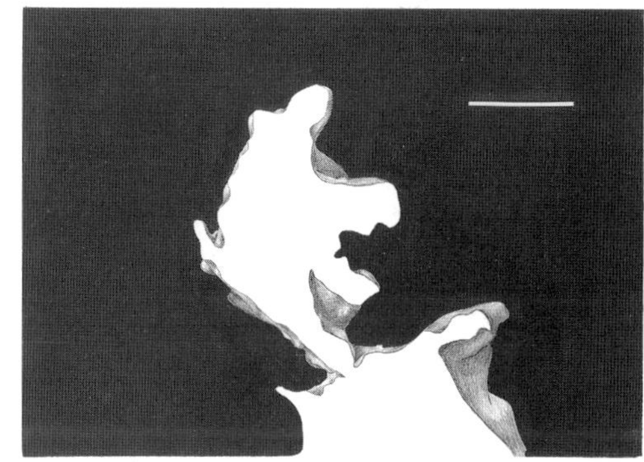

Fig 64b Left half of same primordium, lateral view. Scale: 250 μm.

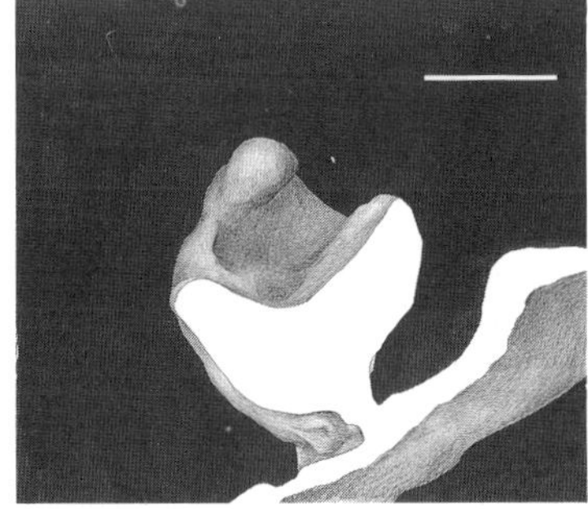

Fig 65a The same fetus (64 mm). Sagittally sectioned right primordium m^1. Right half, medial view. Scale: 250 μm.

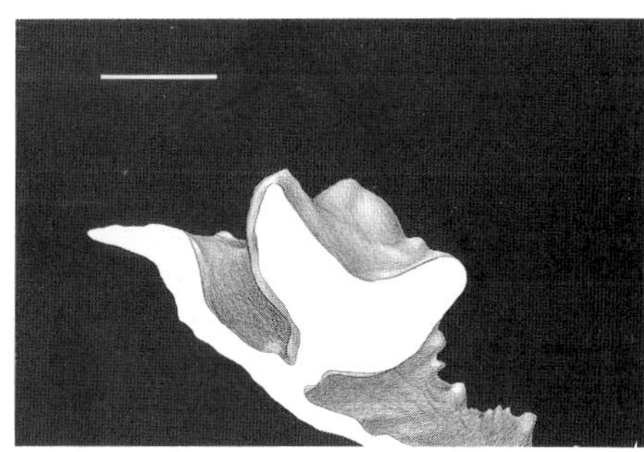

Fig 65b Left half of same primordium, lateral view. Scale: 250 μm.

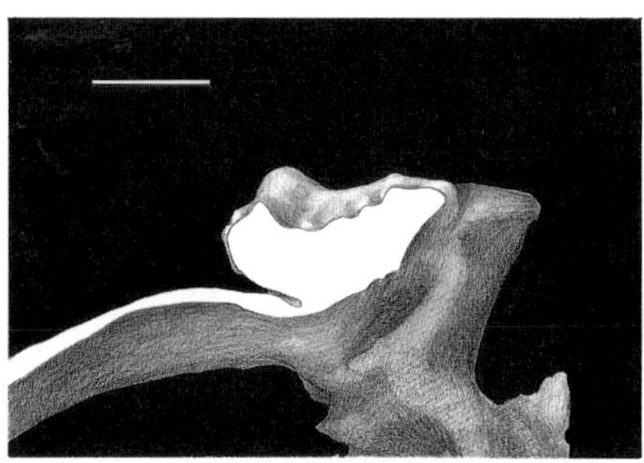

Fig 66a The same fetus (64 mm). Sagittally sectioned right primordium m^2. Right half, medial view. Scale: 250 μm.

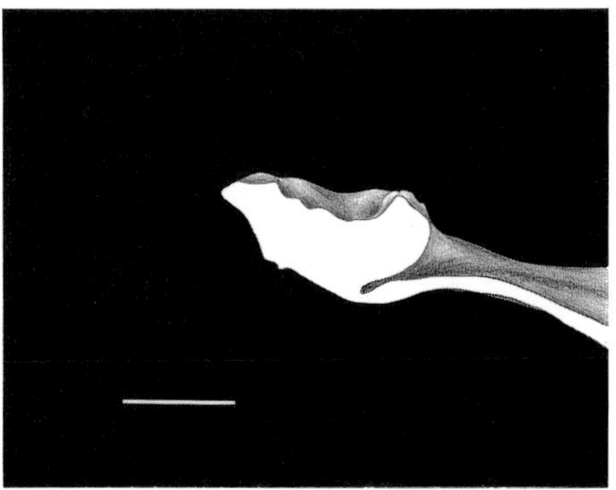

Fig 66b Left half of same primordium, lateral view. Scale: 250 μm.

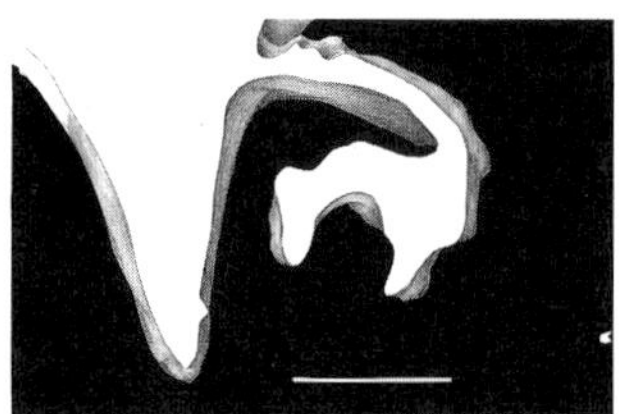

Fig 67a The same fetus (64 mm). Sagittally sectioned right primordium i_1. Right half, medial view. Scale: 250 μm.

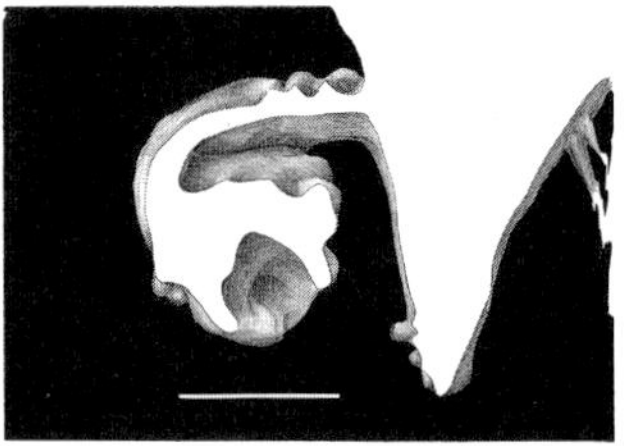

Fig 67b Left half of same primordium, lateral view. Scale: 250 μm.

A sagittal section through the middle of the primordium shows a concave contour of the future inner enamel epithelium of the tooth bell (Fig 71).

As with the primordium of the first mandibular molar, this primordium of m_2 extends into the bony groove of the mandible but does not extend as deep as the primordium of m_1. Meckel's cartilage is covered by an extensive bony posteromedial wall of the groove, whereas the anterolateral wall of the bony groove is not as thick. In this region the groove is narrower, but deeper than below the m_1 primordium. The distance between the floor of the groove and the tooth bell m_2 is about 1,065 μm, and the edges of the groove lie at a distance of about 250 μm from either side of the primordium. As for the more anterior region, the inferior alveolar nerve, artery, and vein run through the mandibular groove underneath the primordium of m_2.

Table 2 summarizes the stages of the primordia with lamina, bud, cap, and bell definitions according to Garn and Burdi (1971).

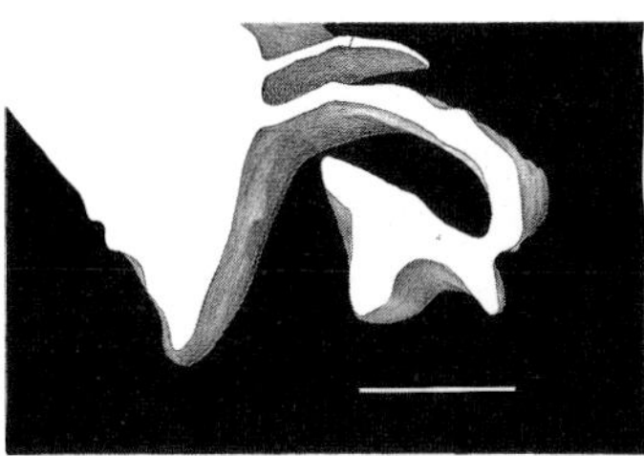

Fig 68a The same fetus (64 mm). Sagittally sectioned right primordium i_2. Right half, medial view. Scale: 250 μm.

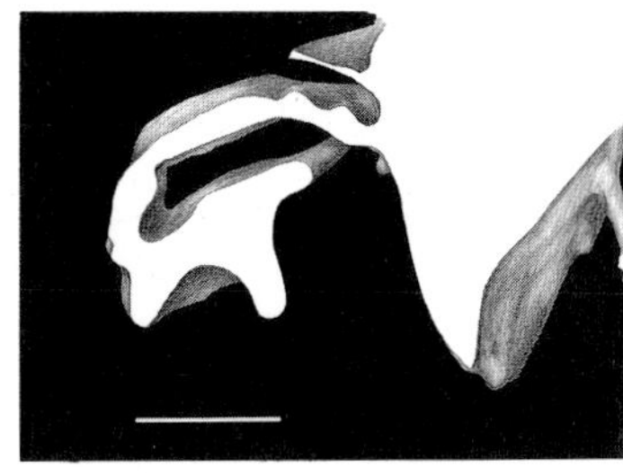

Fig 68b Left half of same primordium, lateral view. Scale: 250 μm.

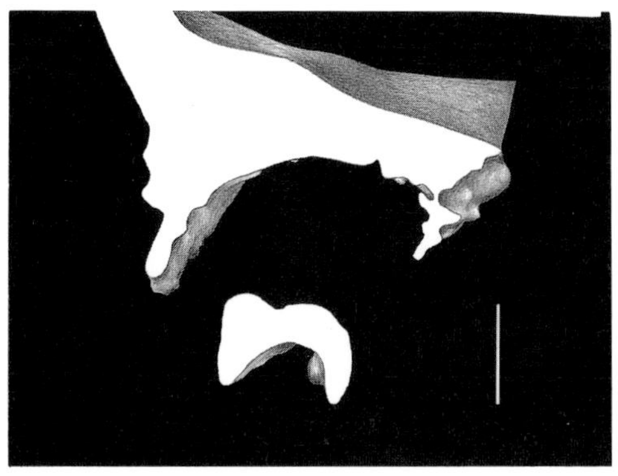

Fig 69a The same fetus (64 mm). Sagittally sectioned right primordium c_1. Right half, medial view. Scale: 250 μm.

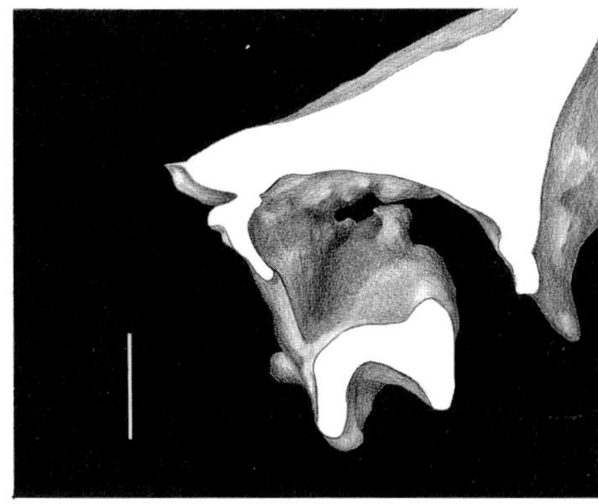

Fig 69b Left half of same primordium, lateral view. Scale: 250 μm.

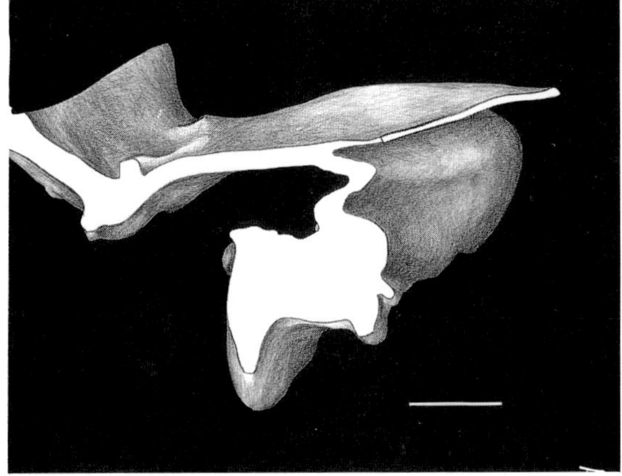

Fig 70a The same fetus (64 mm). Sagittally sectioned right primordium m_1. Right half, medial view. Scale: 250 μm.

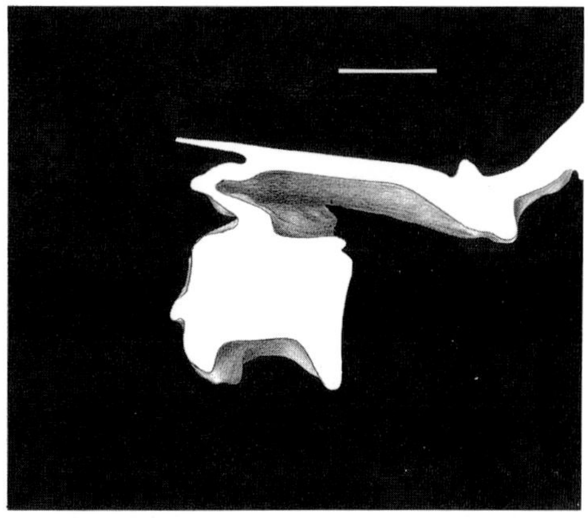

Fig 70b Left half of same primordium, lateral view. Scale: 250 μm.

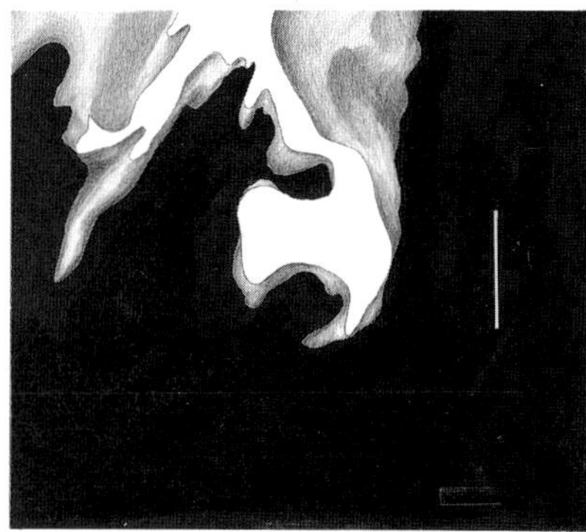

Fig 71a The same fetus (64 mm). Sagittally sectioned right primordium m_2. Right half, medial view. Scale: 250 μm.

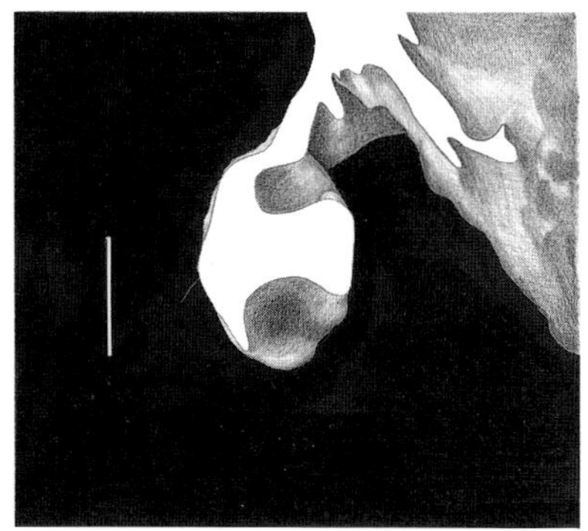

Fig 71b Left half of same primordium, lateral view. Scale: 250 μm.

Table 3 provides a synoptic presentation of the distances between the individual tooth primordia and the bony structures of maxilla and mandible, as well as Meckel's cartilage. (Note: Because the numerical data alone are too rough and subject to certain errors, the reader is referred to previous text and illustrations for a description of the findings.)

Table 2 Summary of the stages of the primordia*

		Maxillary region					Mandibular region				
CRL	Embryo	i^1	i^2	c^1	m^1	m^2	i_1	i_2	c_1	m_1	m_2
17 mm	TON	lamina					lamina				
18 mm	GUS	lamina					lamina				
21 mm	ALI	bud	bud	bud	bud⁻	bud⁻	bud	bud	bud	bud⁻	bud⁻
29 mm	OLL	bud	bud⁻	bud⁺	bud⁻	bud⁻	bud	bud	cap	cap	bud
33 mm	UTE	bud	bud	cap	cap	bud	bud	bud	cap	cap	bud
34 mm	DON	bud	bud	bud⁺	bud	bud	bud	bud	bud	bud⁺	bud
37 mm	DOR	bud	bud	cap	cap⁻	bud	cap⁻	cap⁻	cap	cap⁺	bud
38 mm	HEI	bud	bud	cap	bud	bud	bud	bud	cap	cap	bud
40 mm	PAU	bud⁺	bud⁺	cap	cap	bud	bud	bud	cap	cap	cap⁻
40 mm	ILO	bud	cap⁻	cap	cap⁺	—	bud	bud	cap	cap	—
40 mm	STE	cap	bud	cap	cap	bud	bud	bud	cap	cap	bud
40 mm	QUI	—	—	cap⁺	cap	cap	—	—	cap	cap	cap
45 mm	ERN	cap	bud	cap	cap	cap	bud	bud	cap	cap	bud
47 mm	NIN	cap	cap	cap	cap	cap	cap	cap	cap	cap	cap
53 mm	JOH	cap⁺	cap⁺	bell	bell	bud⁺	cap⁺	cap⁺	bell	cap	cap
56 mm	LIL	cap⁺	cap	bell	bell	bud⁺	cap⁺	cap	bell⁻	bell⁻	bud
60 mm	KAL	cap⁺	cap	bell	bell	cap⁺	bell⁻	cap⁺	bell	bell	cap⁺
64 mm	VER	bell⁻	cap⁺	bell⁻	bell	cap⁺	bell	bell⁻	bell	bell	bell⁻

* Staging of the tooth primordia (lamina, bud, cap, bell) was carried out in accordance with Garn and Burdi (1971). A minus (–) denotes an early, and a plus (+) denotes a later phase within the stages. A long dash indicates that the primordium was not preserved enough to enable staging from the section.

Table 3 Distance in µm between primordia and surrounding structures (bone and Meckel's cartilage)*

		Maxillary region					Mandibular region				
CRL	Embryo	i^1	i^2	c^1	m^1	m^2	i_1	i_2	c_1	m_1	m_2
18 mm	GUS	60					60				
21 mm	ALI	60-80					60-80				
37 mm	DOR	100	90	40-200	100	>200	40 (CM)	60-100	35	250 300	310 (mnd)
47 mm	NIN	100	30-70	50-60	150 200	500	125 (CM)	50 (CM)	120 270	250 800	470 (CM)
64 mm	VER	160 300	130 990	90-530	140 380 540	540	65-85 (mnd) 130 (CM)	110 120 (mnd) 360 (CM)	120 430	100 870	250 1065

* Because bony extensions do not usually lie at a constant distance from the primordium they embrace, minimum and maximum values have been given in most cases. In some cases where bone is found in the sulcus between primordium and vestibular lamina, the minor value refers to the distance between this bone the lamina. Key: (mnd) *mandible;* (CM) *Meckel's cartilage.*

4 Discussion

4.1 Thickening and invagination of the oral epithelium

Invagination of the oral epithelium and formation of the dental and vestibular laminae begins with locally circumscribed alteration of the shape of the cells (Tonge 1960, 1967, 1969). The cuboid epithelial cells become narrow and columnar, causing an initial thickening of the epithelium. There are conflicting data concerning the onset of the thickening of the oral epithelium: the first swelling of the oral epithelium was found by Ooe (1958) in embryos as small as 8 to 9 mm CRL. Ahrens (1913a) describes the first thickening in an embryo of 11 mm CRL. Röse (1893) found epithelial thickenings in embryos of 11 to 14 mm CRL, but he interpreted them as primordia of rudimentary reptile teeth, and he believed, the initiation of the development of the dental lamina starts at a larger stage. According to Orban (1928, 1953), the epithelial thickening begins in an embryo of 13.4 mm CRL, according to Meyer (1951) in embryos of 11 to 14 mm CRL, and according to Norberg (1929) in an embryo of 15 mm CRL.

The extension of these epithelial thickenings, the so-called odontogenic areas (Tonge 1960), is limited to some single islands in an embryo of 28 days of age (Nery et al 1970). In the mandibular region, the invagination of the oral epithelium begins in embryos of 8 to 9 mm CRL (Ooe 1958), at first laterally in the future molar region and later in the anterior region. A continuous lamina can be found in embryos of 15 to 17 mm CRL (Ooe 1958). In the maxillary region there are separate epithelial thickenings on the globular process and on the two maxillary protrusions. They become confluent only after a merging of the lateral nasal prominence with the maxillary prominence, forming a continuous invagination crossing the midfacial region (Ooe 1958). Whereas Hamilton and Mossmann (1972) are convinced that the thickening of the epithelium is due to an increased number of cell divisions in the center of the thickening, Blechschmidt (1955) could not find higher mitotic activity in the epithelium of the incipient dental lamina. The thickening and invagination of this "bandlike placode," (Blechschmidt 1955) which takes place earlier in the mandibular than in the maxillary region, is seen to be a result of the spatial impediment in connection with the development of the upper and lower lips (Röse 1892a, Preuss 1953, Blechschmidt 1955, 1960). The upper and lower lips increase in size, roll in, and bend sharply at their transition into the antilabial folds (Blechschmidt 1960). In these same sharp bends, the invagination of the oral epithelium is initiated. Further subdivision leads to the formation of the dental and vestibular laminae.

According to McLoughlin (1963), Rawles (1963), and Kollar (1972), the mesenchyme underneath the epithelium is condensed prior to epithelial thickening, whereas Blechschmidt (1948), Steding (1967), and Jacob (1970) generally consider mesenchymal condensation a consequence of epithelial thickening.

4.2 Laminar stage

4.2.1 Pattern of invagination of vestibular and dental laminae

There have been contradictory views as to whether the dental and vestibular laminae arise as two separate foldings of the oral epithelium or whether they are subdivisions of a common invagination: Bolk (1911), Norberg (1929), Schour (1929), McMurrich (1912), Florian and Frankenberger

(1936), as well as Orban (1953) and Tonge (1960, 1969), are convinced that dental and vestibular laminae are two separate formations that invaginate into the underlying mesenchyme. This view contrasts with that of Röse (1891), Widdowson (1948), Plackova (1963), Mjör and Pindborg (1973), and Scott and Symons (1974), who are certain that dental and vestibular laminae develop from a common epithelial invagination.

In histologic studies, depending on the direction of the section plane, there will be different outlines of the invaginated structure, which may explain the different statements concerning this issue. Plackova (1963), well aware of the projection error in two-dimensional histology, commenced the description of her study of the dental lamina with a sketch to illustrate the projection phenomenon. She did her study, however, without three-dimensional reconstructions, which of course would have elucidated the problem.

This study using three-dimensional reconstruction confirms the descriptions of Meyer (1951) and Schroeder (1987) and solves the contradiction. The invagination of the dental and the vestibular lamina follows both patterns: in the *anterior* region vestibular and dental laminae are subdivisions from a common thickened epithelial basis, while in the *posterior* region vestibular and dental laminae are clearly discernible as two single invaginations of the oral epithelium. The reconstruction of the 18-mm embryo of this study shows how the dental and vestibular laminae arise from their common epithelial ledge. Particularly in the mandibular region, the separation of the two epithelial subdivisions is just beginning and is indicated by a discontinuous shallow furrow of the invaginated epithelial band. Toward the lateral region, the vestibular lamina levels out in this early embryological stage and is no longer visible in the posterior region. Only reconstructions of later stages, of embryos of 33 mm and of 47 mm CRL, show a deep furrow severing the two laminae in the posterior region. Thus, here one may well speak of two separate invaginations of the oral epithelium, provided that the oral epithelium between the two laminae maintains its normal thickness. Although the vestibular lamina of the posterior region is the continuous extension of that of the anterior region, it invaginates later and clearly further laterally in older fetuses. The findings lead to the conclusion that the invagination proceeds from an anterior to a posterior direction.

There are hints that some of the epithelial invaginations may be only temporary formations. Thus, in the fetus of 47 mm CRL there was an invagination of the oral epithelium medially from the primordium of m_2. This epithelial folding was much more defined than the vestibular lamina of this region, which showed only slight swellings of the oral epithelium (Fig 34). In an older fetus (64 mm CRL) a clear vestibular lamina has formed lateral to the primordium of m_2, whereas the epithelium in the region medial to m_2 has flattened (Fig 52).

4.2.2 *Nebenleiste* and prelacteal lamina

In some cases (for example, Fig 39) an additional folding of the epithelium can be found between the tooth primordium and the vestibular lamina. Bolk (1913) and Ahrens (1913 a) call this the *Nebenleiste*, Bolk (1913) interpreting it as a rudiment of the vestibular lamina of reptiles.

Highly polemic arguments were exchanged by Adloff (1909, 1913 a, 1913 b, 1914) and Ahrens (1913 b) concerning the so-called prelacteal lamina. This supposedly was an additional epithelial lamina that should have indicated a dentition prior to the first dentition. Adloff (1909, 1913 a, 1913 b, 1914) vehemently maintained that the additional invaginations of the epithelium found by him represent the existence of a prelacteal lamina of man as well as of other species.

The findings of the present study confirm the *observations* of additional epithelial foldings in some of the embryos of our collection. Several additional invaginations of the vestibular lamina were found: some were more toward the dental primordium, and in addition, secondary foldings of the vestibular lamina could be found in the more anterior region. These extended for a short distance of 60 μm as well as for a longer distance of 500 μm (Radlanski and Jäger 1991 a). The reconstructions clearly reveal, however, that these additional foldings arise from the *vestibular* lamina, and not from the *dental* lamina. Morphologically, therefore, it may be concluded that these foldings should not be considered precursors of dental primordia. Histochemical or genetic analysis of cellular material from these foldings may further elucidate this question.

Bolk's (1913) view of the *Nebenleiste* and Adloff's (1909, 1913 a, 1913 b, 1914) conclusion regarding the prelacteal lamina both attribute these formations as remnants of an additional independent dentition. Some contemporaries (Röse 1895, Kükenthal 1914) adopted their opinion, but Ahrens (1913 a) strictly opposed it; he simply called these formations what they are: additional invaginations. A basic question arises here: can an epithelial folding, which does not develop any further than the stage of lamina, be considered to be *dentogenous* organ, although teeth have never been observed developing from such formations? Following the teleologic view, some claim that any formation (in this case, a folded one) must have a meaning, a function, or a purpose (Peter 1920) even if it is as yet unknown. Thus, it can be understood why, from the existence of such epithelial foldings, it was concluded to remnants of former primordia of ancestors, or to first signs of future organs yet to evolve (de Beer 1951). It was particularly after the publication of Haeckel's law of biogenetics in 1874 that most people, except Ahrens (1913 a), usually were not satisfied with the pure *finding* that these invaginated formations were in the first instance nothing but foldings of the epithelium. Blechschmidt (1948, 1960), incorporating the ideas of His (1874), refuted the law of biogenetics by detailed and systematic findings and set his *Genetisches Grundgesetz*[7] (Blechschmidt 1964) against it. In this way he detached embryology from its historical mix-ups, and stated that the meaning of foldings that arise during morphogenesis must be understood only from the developmental movements of the growing fetus; he saw no way in which the individual's historical (phylogenetic) background could play a morphogenetically active influence.[8]

7. Literally translated *Genetisches Grundgesetz* would mean *basic genetic law*, and it would imply a basic genetic control of development. Those who study Blechschmidt's attitude toward genetic activity (*Mechanische Genwirkungen*, Blechschmidt 1948), however, would not be satisfied with this translation. Blechschmidt, not denying the genes at all (personal communication, March 25, 1985), attributes a more reactive role to the genetic code in order to cope with developmental changes of form and to maintain metabolic activity. So *genetic* is meant more in the sense of *creative*. A more modern view is given in *Anatomie und Ontogenese des Menschen* (Blechschmidt 1978).
8. It is interesting to see how differently this point of view was accepted by contemporary anatomists: Elze's (1949/50) book review concerning *Mechanische Genwirkungen* (Blechschmidt 1948) sounds quite affirmative, whereas Starck (1949) defends the phylogenetic-embryological point of view.

This is not the place to extend this discussion any further. However, it should be mentioned at least that Ahrens (1913 b) found the same epithelial foldings as Adloff (1909, 1913 a, 1913 b, 1914), but Ahrens (1913 b) constructed solid models from serial sections and did not find any structures that developed beyond the shape of epithelial folds. He reproached Adloff, who did not even use *serial* sections, with the inadmissibility of his interpretations to this problem after examining only one single section.

4.2.3 Outline of the dental lamina

In his reconstructions of early dental laminae, Ooe (1958) showed that the bulge facing the mesenchyme has a wavy contour as soon as invagination has formed. The reconstructions of the embryos of 18 mm CRL and 21 mm CRL in this study confirm his finding. The dental lamina is neither invaginated to constant depth, nor is it of constant thickness, as it is shown very schematically (probably for didactic reasons) in some textbooks (Eidmann 1923, Meyer 1951, Hamilton and Mossmann 1972). The early dental lamina has a variable contour in different regions. It is not known whether there is a *regularity* in the variability of the wavy contour of the dental lamina in the sense that certain bulging patterns could be related to a specific primordial region. This might answer the question whether the different shapes from bud to bud may have their origin in typical patterns of variation of early epithelial bulges of the dental lamina. More reconstructions of early dental laminae are required to resolve this question.

4.3 Bud stage

Aside from singular observations of deviation in the number of teeth (Ooe 1971), usually five distinct swellings of the dental lamina, the tooth buds, arise per quadrant. Formation of buds is reported to occur earlier in the mandibular region than in the maxillary region. In addition, the more anterior primordia usually develop ahead of the posterior primordia (Burdi et al 1970).
It is not known what triggers the circumscribed regional thickening of the dental lamina. From the regularity in the locations of buds, the existence of

morphogenetic fields was concluded (Butler 1939, Glasstone 1963, Garn et al 1965, Miller 1969, van Valen 1970, Garn and Burdi 1971, Thiebold et al 1974). Further, a source of oscillation was assumed to exist at the mesial end of the jaw, producing some kind of waves running along the dental lamina and stimulating competent cells to perform the transition from the lamina stage to the bud stage (Kieser 1984). Gaunt (1959) concludes there are possible inductive potentials from the proximity between early blood vessels and the dental lamina. Similar processes leading to initiation of bud formation, provoked by early nerve endings, are assumed by Pearson (1977) and by Kollar and Lumsden (1978).

To the discussion and interpretation of the findings there may be added another assumption, namely that deduced from the topographic arrangement of the perioral structures. The reconstruction of the 21-mm embryo (Figs 6 to 8) leads to the following hypothesis: in the bud stage the dental lamina achieves a spatial relation with its surrounding structures so that the spatial impediment of the expanding dental epithelium may be a cause for differential bulging and for the formation of buds (Radlanski et al 1988a). Steding (1967) showed that thickening of growing epithelium occurs as a consequence of spatial impediment from ring implants. He suggests that formation of tooth buds may be a result of the same principle.

Thus, following formation of the dental lamina by invagination of the epithelium, mitotic activity in the epithelium continues as it grows inward. A spatial impediment is obviously present at the distal ends of the dental lamina and is due to Meckel's cartilage and the ascendent ramus of the early mandible. Therefore, in this region an increasing number of cells may lead to a compression and bulging of the dental lamina. During bulging, cell shape is altered either to narrow and cylindrical or to a wedge-shaped outline (Radlanski et al 1989). It was Blechschmidt (1948, 1960) who showed that such epithelia with wedge-shaped cells generally are developed in regions that are characterized by spatial impediment. These wedge-shaped epithelia are precursors for the primordia of many other organs, for example, glands, hair follicles, or the buds of the early limbs.

There is another fact that may support the idea that mechanical factors are of importance: the reconstruction in Fig 7 shows that the buds protrude in a *lingual* direction, and not, as described by Meyer (1951), in a *vestibular* direction. The bent dental lamina, while continuously growing, therefore suffers more compression at its lingual (concave) side, which leads to bulging and protrusion of the buds.

For the human primary dentition we find a constant number of five such areas per quadrant. This numerical constancy can be see to be a result of the unique material properties of this specific kind of epithelial cells (for example, stiffness of the epithelial band, mutual adhesion of cell membranes, elasticity of cellular matrix), and of the availability of space for this epithelial formation. Later, just enough space remains to allow the dental lamina to form the primordia for the permanent dentition. If we could experimentally extend the distal end of the dental lamina we would expect additional density centers and, thus, an increased number of tooth buds. Here, more embryological research focusing on comparative anatomy should be carried out to elucidate the spatial relationships in representatives of various species with different numbers of teeth.

In addition, more research must be carried out to determine why tooth buds with subsequent stages are formed from the epithelial thickenings of the dental lamina. For the further development of tooth germs, adaequate space for mitotic activity must be regained. This might be accomplished by further growth of the surrounding structures (eg, growth of Meckel's cartilage, and possibly the descent of the heart), which counteract the original spatial restriction.

Although Ooe (1956, 1958, 1959, 1981) has published a great number of reconstructions of tooth buds, a comprehensive comparison of the different form of the buds has not yet been undertaken. Because the initial question is whether there are differences of gestalt between the tooth primordia, one should start comparative evaluations as early as the bud stage, if not the lamina stage. The findings of this study derived from the reconstructions of the bud stage show clear early differences: the primordia of i_1 in the 21-mm and in the 28-mm embryo, for example, are clearly flat and extend more into mesiodistal direction. The buds of i_2 and the maxillary primordia of the incisors and the canines are, in contrast, more rounded. The mandibular molar primordia are rather oval, with their greatest diameter parallel to the dental lamina.

These findings, based more or less on individual cases, are not sufficient to deduce regularities between typical shapes of tooth primordia and their position in the arch. This, however, would be necessary if one wanted to determine whether all primordia arise from standardized, identical buds, and only in later stages differentiate into the different typical teeth, or whether the typical differences of the adult teeth can be traced back into earliest stages. A more systematic and thorough examination of many more cases will have to be carried out.

Ooe (1958) states that the primordia obtain different distances within the dental arch. This can be seen in his figures, too. In contrast, the reconstructions of this study always show a uniform distance between each other (an exception is the lesser distance between the right and left primordium i_1 in the 21-mm embryo). There are general differences, however, between the mandibular and the maxillary region: the interprimordial distances are greater in the maxillary region. This study shows that it is only in later stages of development, in the late cap stage and in the early bell stage, that different distances are found between the tooth primordia, so then accordance is gained back to Ooe (1956, 1981).

4.4 Cap stage

The developmental sequence after which the tooth primordia reach the cap stage in the embryos of this study agrees with the data of Garn and Burdi (1971), and Butler (1989).[9] Usually the primordia of the canine and the first molar (of the primary dentition) are the first dental primordia to reach the cap stage. However, as these authors pointed out, extreme deviations from this developmental scheme can be found. Table 2 of this study corroborates their findings and shows that dental maturity and body size do not necessarily match in every case. This fact is, by the way, well known from clinical experience because shedding of teeth may occur within a wider age range.

In addition, there is variability regarding the size of the primordia and their development stages. In the 47-mm fetus, all primordia are further developed than in the 37-mm fetus. The buds and the early caps of the 37-mm fetus, however, are already about the same size as the later caps of the 47-mm fetus. This finding, again, matches the clinically well-known, wide range of tooth size in interindividual comparison. Further, in these early stages it can clearly be shown that the primordia of the maxillary incisors are larger than those of the mandibular incisors, although the latter are further developed. This difference is more obvious in the 64-mm fetus.

In some cases typical differences of gestalt and developmental maturity between the different primordia are maintained during the transition from the bud stage to the cap stage: the mandibular caps i_1 and i_2 are clearly oval in mesiodistal direction in the 37-mm fetus, as is the case with the same buds of the 21-mm embryo. The canine primordium of the 29-mm embryo was slightly advanced in development, as in the 37-mm fetus. The early cap of m_1 remains as oval in mesiodistal direction in the 37-mm fetus as in the 29-mm embryo. The primordia m^1 and m^2 of the 29-mm embryo are discernible only as early epithelial protrusions, so a meaningful comparison with the gestalt of the older primordia of the 37-mm fetus is not possible at this stage. Between 29 and 37 mm CRL the primordium m_2 did not essentially change its form, only its position: the bud m_2, which is located exactly at the distal end of the dental lamina in the 37-mm fetus, is located about 50 μm anterior to its distal end in the younger embryo of 29 mm CRL. The late buds i^1 and i^2 of the 37-mm fetus maintained the round outline that they had in the 21-mm embryo.

The form of a completed tooth crown is very much dependent on the extension and the developmental movements of the inner enamel epithelium, the cells of which will develop into ameloblasts (Schroeder 1982, Schumacher et al 1990). It may be supposed that the potential developmental movements of the inner enamel epithelium are to a certain extent influenced by the development of the outer epithelium of the tooth primordium. It would thus seem to be important to describe not only the outer aspect of the cap, but the aspect facing the mesenchymal papilla as well. For this reason, the reconstructions are depicted from medial and lateral views, supplemented by views from an obliquely caudal or cranial direction. In this way the shallow concavities of the caps can be evaluated.

9. Personal communication, June 6, 1989.

In addition, the outlines of the caps were described from a vertical ("occlusal") view, enabling comparisons with the occlusal outline of the completed tooth.

In the stage of the late caps, represented here by the reconstruction of the 47-mm fetus, differences between the primordia regarding their gestalt become more obvious than in earlier stages. Now some of the primordia clearly possess characteristics of the completed teeth: the caps i^1 and i^2 are clearly flat in a mesiodistal direction, the cap c^1 has a more triangular outline, if seen from a cranial direction. The primordium m^1 resembles a rectangle, and it is, in addition, the largest primordium of this embryo. The cap m^2 is more flat and possesses a trapezoidal outline. Like the maxillary primordia just described, the mandibular primordia have developed recognizable characteristic features. Thus, the incisal primordium i_1 is oval if seen from a caudal direction, whereas i_2 still is rounder in shape. The canine primordium is almost triangular, similar to the maxillary primordium. The outline of the primordium of the first primary mandibular molar resembles almost an oblong pentagon, and the primordium m_2 has a rather rhombic outline.

Besides the differences between those parts of the tooth primordia directly involved in dental morphogenesis, there exist different morphological features when attention is focused on those parts of the primordia that face the general dental lamina. Because a lateral enamel lamina (Bolk 1913) arises to run from every primordium in a more or less lateral direction toward the general dental lamina, there are also formed deeper enamel niches (Bolk 1913) and more shallow enamel troughs (Meyer 1951). The niche and trough are confined by the tooth primordium itself, by the lateral enamel lamina, and by the general dental lamina. Meyer (1951) reports that the more funnel-shaped enamel niche in all primordia can be found in a distal direction, with the exception of the first primary molar primordium, in which the enamel niche points in a mesial direction. The more shallow enamel trough is usually located at the mesial aspect of the primordium, but for the case of the first primary molars, it is, according to Meyer (1951), more shallow in a distal direction and here is therefore called enamel *trough*. Meyer (1951) reports that the situation concerning the direction of enamel niche and enamel trough in the primordia of the second primary molars is similar to that in the primordia of the anterior teeth.

The reconstructions of this study regarding the different position and depth of the deeper enamel niche and the more shallow enamel trough confirm the descriptions of Meyer (1951), principally for incisor and canine primordia. For the molar primordia, however, agreement with Meyer (1951) could not be found in every case: in the cap stage of m_2, the deeper, funnel-shaped cave is located mesially and not distally. In m_1, both mesial and distal niches are of almost the same depth, and in m^2, the excavation is deeper mesially. Only concerning m^1 is there agreement with Meyer (1951), who finds the deeper niche mesially.

Although the primordium and the lateral enamel lamina are tightly associated in the cap stage, the present data are insufficient to deduce a possible morphogenetic potential whereby the lateral enamel lamina could influence the shape of the tooth primordium. It might be necessary to devote more attention to this part of the primordium in another study.

Next to all these differences there is one common feature possessed by all the caps: they all open in a distal direction, although to different extents. This is due to the marginal bulging, which is not as high or is even missing in certain distal regions of the caps. In his graphic reconstructions of molar primordia, Turner (1959, 1967) found that formation of the enamel organ proceeds mesiodistally and that the growth increase of the epithelium is oriented preferably in a horizontal direction. Only later does the epithelium also bulge into the depth at the distal margin, also distally.

In examining the reconstructions of Meyer (1951) it must be noticed that in his drawings the incisor primordia of similar stages show a greater diameter in vestibulo-oral direction. This is in contrast to the findings of this study.

There are no comparable descriptions in the literature referring to the spatial arrangement of the early dental primordia and their neighboring structures (maxilla, mandible, Meckel's cartilage), as they can be observed in the present reconstructions of the 37-mm and the 47-mm fetus. For later stages, there are data from the work of Gantz (1922), who used an oil-clearing method to show the position of the tooth germs within the mandibles of fetuses. However, his youngest specimen had already reached 110 mm CRL. Norberg (1933) reconstructed the development of the alveolar compartments, starting with a fetus of 139 mm CRL. Much later stages were studied by Baume (1955) and by Böcker and Becker (1965), who discuss the mutual influences between the topogenesis of dental primordia and their surrounding bony structures. As can be seen, these studies refer to fetuses that are much older than the oldest specimens of the present study.

Looking at the reconstruction of the 47-mm fetus and considering the different forms of the dental primordia and their spatial relationships to the neighboring structures (bone and Meckel's cartilage), it may be concluded that in this stage the proximity between dental primordia and harder structures can no longer play a role in shaping the primordia. Whereas in the bud stage spatial impediments, leading to the formation of the protrusions of the dental lamina, could be a factor, there is no hint of similar effects exerted on the dental primordia by the surrounding structures in the cap stage. The only question that does arise in this connection is whether there is an interdependence between the flat shape of the primordia i_1 of the 37-mm fetus and its position cranial to the protruding anterior end of Meckel's cartilage: the mesenchymal cells surrounding the anterior part of Meckel's cartilage are flattened and show a characteristic orientation, from which a growth expansion of the cartilage structure can be concluded. However, during further development, the distance from i_1 to Meckel's cartilage increases as a result of the general increase in vertical facial dimension.

It is therefore still questionable whether an important mechanical contribution to the flatness of the primordia i_1 can be derived by the proximity of Meckel's cartilage. Not only are the primordia i_1 (which are so close to Meckel's cartilage in the 21-mm and the 37-mm fetus) so flat, but the primordia i_2, which are further away from Meckel's cartilage in every stage, also undergo a transition from round to flat. In addition, the maxillary incisor primordia of the 37-mm fetus are almost well rounded, whereas in the 47-mm fetus they are typically flattened in the direction of the future incisal edge. The reconstructions of the 47-mm fetus do not offer any hint of spatial impediment in vestibulo-oral direction, which may correlate with this flattening of the dental epithelium. A study is in progress to elucidate whether flattening of the incisal primordia may be a consequence of a transversal development of the dental lamina arch mediated by the transversal development of the face and of the nasal capsule and Meckel's cartilage in particular.

4.5 Bell stage

4.5.1 Comparative anatomy of the primordia in the bell stage

The reconstructions of this study showing the primordia in the stage of the early bells make it easier to understand the differences between the primordia. Perhaps this is due to the fact that at this stage the epithelial formations resemble more and more the shapes of the completed teeth as known from clinical experience.

When the tooth primordia have reached the early bell stage, the first foldings of the inner enamel epithelium have developed. These foldings may be interpreted as the first sings of the future typical occlusal pattern.

As mentioned, it is obvious that teeth of different shape and form can be traced back to epithelial primordia, which must have an accordingly different shape and form. This is particularly true for the future inner enamel epithelium, which later will secrete the enamel matrix; the outer gestalt of the outer enamel epithelium might as well be of importance, since the outer gestalt of the dental primordium functions as a limitation for the expansion of the inner enamel epithelium. However, detailed differences over the various stages have not yet been presented in a sufficiently comprehensive way. It was Ahrens (1913 a)who first mentioned this fact, and he did supply some reconstruction models. However, his published models represent only a limited selection of primordia, and therefore a regional comparison between the primordia within the same dental arch was not possible. From his findings, he concludes that in the earlier bud and cap stages it is, concerning the form, not yet possible to distinguish the primordium of an incisor from that of a molar. Only in the later bell stage does he supply distinct descriptions of development of the different primordia. For the incisors he states, "As can be seen, one can easily deduce the form of the completed incisor's crown from the form of the primordium of this stage. The enamel organ represents, so to speak, the casting mold for the incisor crown." [10] He does not describe this development of form by means of reconstruction models but with histologic sections; the typical contour of the gestalt of the incisor with the sharp incisal edge and the lingual tubercle is indeed clearly visible. There is no shortage of demonstrations like these: a considerable number of them are also found in Meyer (1951), who also describes the development of the anterior teeth separately from the molars. However, as discussed above, what is really needed here are three-dimensional reconstructions, which enable us to perform a longitudinal and an intraindividual regional comparison.

As mentioned, Ahrens (1913a) does not distinguish between the development of primordia in the bud, cap, and early bell stage. Only for the later bell stages, in subsequent parts of his study, does he work out the difference of gestalt between the primordia of anterior and lateral teeth, too. Here he now offers very distinct descriptions, exemplified by detailed wax-plate reconstructions. In principle these findings corroborate my reconstructions of the early bell stage (cf Fig 70), but the comparison is not quite appropriate. Ahrens (1913a) demonstrates the development using the example of a *permanent* molar; the development of the primary molars is mentioned only incidentally.

In the incisor primordia, in i_1 more clearly than in i^1 the contour of the inner enamel epithelium is developed in such a characteristic way that the early bell stage can be called, as Ahrens (1913a) called it, the casting mold of the completed tooth. [11] Here my findings corroborate the temporal data given by Nomata (1964), who also found the first sharp, incisal-edge-like bend of the epithelial contour of i_1 in a fetus of 64 mm CRL. A contour that may correspond to the lingual tubercle was found by him in fetuses of 78 and 84 mm CRL. My findings show a tuberculum-like bend already indicated in the primordium i_1 in the 64-mm fetus (Fig 67). Although the deposition of enamel will alter the shape of the crown, the typical contour of an incisor is clearly recognizable in this stage. Further research, perhaps with some marking technique, must show to what extent cellular material forming these characteristic bends retains responsibility for them while moving into the periphery during enamel matrix deposition. The primordia of the maxillary and mandibular second primary incisors have not yet developed to the same extent and do not reveal such a contour.

The canine primordia, again, are different from the incisal primordia, because their cross section is neither ellipsoid nor oval but more round or triangular. In sagittal section, the canine primordia show barely any difference to the contour of the inner enamel epithelium of the primordia of i^1.

Finally, the molar primordia, particularly those of the first molars, anticipate the more rectangular outline of the completed tooth. A typical *relief* cannot yet be found in the primordia of the maxillary molars, but possibly in the primordium of the mandibular first primary molar: here, in sagittal section, it is possible to clearly distinguish two separate concavities of the epithelial contour, and in between a slight caudal protrusion (Fig 70).

According to Nomata (1964), invaginations of the epithelium that can be clearly coordinated to single cusps do not arise before the fetus has reached a size of 170 to 180 mm CRL. The first formations of an occlusal relief of the inner enamel epithelium of the tooth bell of m_1, however, are highly visible in the 64-mm fetus of this study (Fig 70). These first indications of epithelial foldings may be the initial conditions for further formation of the typical molar occlusal cusp and fissure pattern.

4.5.2 Assumptions concerning cusp formation

If we ask for the causes of cusp formation, we find an abundance of different and sometimes contradictory concepts in the literature.

The observation that different teeth can be dissected into several single elements of the same contour triggered many efforts to solve the question concerning the principle of tooth formation. From the fact that molars bear several cusps in anterioposterior as well as in buccolingual direction, Cope (1871) concluded that a "law of repeti-

10. Translated by the author. German original: *"Wie man sieht, kann man aus der Form des Schmelzorgans in diesem Stadium die Form der fertigen Schneidezahnkrone einfach ableiten. Das Schmelzorgan stellt sozusagen eine Gussform der Schneidezahnkrone dar."* (Ahrens, p 193).

11. It must be remembered, however, that this comparison is not quite correct, because enamel is not poured into this mold-like shell, but it is the secretion product of the moving inner enamel epithelium. In this way, of course, it alters its spatial arrangement by growing and expanding.

tive addition'' was operating. He was convinced that he had found a morphogenetic principle to explain the ontogenesis of teeth, as well as other embryological formations. In my judgment, some of the embryological ideas that Cope developed in his 1871 article have not lost currency today.

Another approach is the theory of concrescence offered by Kükenthal (1892), Röse (1892b), and Schwalbe (1894), with their phylogenetic attempt to explain the evolutionary development of tooth form. According to this theory the occlusal pattern of the molars, which is characterized by numerous cusps, should have its origin in an evolutionary fusion of several single-cusped teeth, as are found, for example, in reptiles. The *Dimertheorie* by Bolk (1911, 1913) is, in principle, another kind of concrescence theory. Here, two primordia of ancestral reptiles are meant to be the basic element for one mammalian molar.

These assumptions are contrasted by the theory of differentiation, represented particularly by the theory of trituberculy of Cope (1883, 1889) and Osborn (1892). Here the homodont reptilian tooth should have changed gradually into a multicusped, tritubercular tooth. Another theory of differentiation is Anthony's (1970) theory of multituberculy, according to which the mammalian molar has differentiated from less complex multicusped ancestral teeth. Today the tritubercular theory of Cope (1883, 1889) and Osborn (1892) is favored by Starck (1982). The theory of concrescence is considered to be outdated because it can no longer be matched with contemporary paleontologic and embryological knowledge (Starck 1982).

At this point the basic question must be considered, whether one can gain any knowledge at all about ontogenetic processes from phylogenetic studies (de Beer 1951). Although it cannot be denied that there is an evolution with continuous change of forms from generation to generation, it must be clearly stated that, from an evolutionary development, the factors active in ontogenetic morphogenesis of the individual cannot be deduced (Meyer 1926, Blechschmidt 1976). The criteria according to which a phylogenetic tree is ''reconstructed'' are mostly of a typologic and historical nature, and experimental proof is impossible. Thus, history cannot be an explanation for questions concerned with individual morphogenesis. Teeth offer excellent opportunity for research for evolutionary biologists because they are such a durable part of the body. However, regarding the just-cited objection (ie, the explanatory value of this kind of research), the findings of phylogenetic studies must be evaluated appropriately (Meyer 1926, Goll 1972, Blechschmidt 1976) when applied to odontogenesis.

From the similarities and variations of the occlusal pattern there were derived an abundance of genetic regularities (Korkhaus 1940, Dahlberg 1945, 1965, Garn et al 1963, 1967, Osborne 1967, Fitzgerald 1969, Müller 1975, Garn 1977, Harzer 1987), which are more or less meant as supplements or contributions to contemporary evolutionary concepts. These studies do not describe biochemical genetic actions, but rather they are detailed descriptions from a comparative anatomic viewpoint. What can be expected from molecular genetics and its efforts to bridge the gap between genetics and morphogenesis is briefly mentioned in the introductory section 1.2.2 of this study.

Another explanatory concept is the morphogenetic field. Because the single teeth are so clearly different and can be characterized as incisors, canines, premolars, and molars, and because they are usually located at specific places within the dental arch, the concept of morphogenetic fields became obvious (Butler 1939). There thus arose descriptions of incisivation, caninization, and molarization fields (Miller 1969, van Valen 1970, Thiebold et al 1974). It is a characteristic of fields (Waddington 1956) that their potentials (ie, capacities to develop) are taken over with the tissue when transplantations are performed (Glasstone 1963). The idea of a ''field,'' however, is rather conceptual than technical (Goodwin and Cohen 1969), and so the existence of a field cannot be determined independently from morphogenetic processes taking place therein. The same objection can be made for Blechschmidt's (1948, 1960, 1978) ''metabolic fields'': actions like contusion, condensation, cuneation, dilation, detraction, and distusion can well be deduced in the respected fields from alterations at a histologic and micromorphological level. However, physical measurements to evaluate the proposed different forces have not yet been performed successfully independently from what happens to the tissue within the ''fields.''

The idea that tooth form (gestalt) may be considered to be composed of structural repetition of single elements needs further discussion. The concept of serial repetition of structural elements forming anatomic units is called *merism* according to Bateson (1894). In addition to the previously mentioned law of repetitive addition (Cope 1871), there are other findings that deserve mention in this context. Cope (1871) considered the cusps the basic element of molars; Stein (1934) discussed Gregory's (1934) "polyisomerism" (presence of similar parts, isomeres, in different teeth of the same dentition); and Butler carries his own views on dental merism further in his 1967 paper. d'Eternod (1911) stated that the premolar of the human dentition can be interpreted as a general basic element of the human tooth: multiplied in a distal direction, it represents molars, and in a mesial direction, it can be found in the incisors and canines, when the oral cusp is thought to be reduced. Kubein-Meesenburg et al (1986) show that the palatal concavity in a sagittal section of a maxillary incisor matches the slope of the cusp of a premolar sectioned the same way. This observation is significant for the biomechanics of occlusal function (Kubein-Meesenburg et al 1988 a, b).

Next to a practical, functional, gnathologic interpretation, and next to genetic and phylogenetic speculations, dental merism (in the sense that teeth look as if composed from single cusps and that identical contours can be found at different teeth) can be explained on an embryological basis. In general, when glands or lung alveolae develop, it can be observed that the size of the gland bud is limited. Further growth leads rather to the formation of two buds (dichotomous division) and not to the formation of a single larger bud (Blechschmidt 1960). There seems to be a certain "largest single unit." Accordingly, premolars are definitely smaller than molars, and they usually have only two cusps. Molars, being larger, have four or more cusps.[12] It is important to note that the size of the cusps does not correspond to the overall size discrepancy between premolars and molars; the size of the molar cusps is similar to that of the premolar cusps, but their number is higher; and usually it is not the case that molars are just enlarged premolars with correspondingly larger cusps. In supernumerary teeth, too, we find only one cusp when they are small, but as soon as they exceed a certain size they are bicuspid (Butler 1967).

Formation of enamel cusps has its origin in the folding pattern of the inner enamel epithelium. During further tooth development enamel matrix is deposited while the ameloblasts move in an occlusal direction, and dentin is secreted by the odontoblasts, which move toward the dental pulp. The primary status of the folded inner enamel epithelium is conserved as the dentinoenamel junction within the tooth. The enamel mantle of the tooth is of variable thickness, so the initial folding pattern of the inner enamel epithelium is not so clearly visible at the occlusal surface of the molars.

It may be speculated that the same basic principles of folding are applicable for the inner enamel epithelium as were found in glands or lung alveolae (as mentioned above). Thus, a hypothesis may be developed for the formation of an occlusal relief with cusps of almost the same size (Radlanski et al 1988 b). The inner enamel epithelium obtains a specific folding pattern that is dependent on the amount of space to be covered: in larger molar primordia the inner enamel epithelium folds several times, in smaller premolar primordia it folds only twice. The maximal size of a single vault, before it is forced to collapse and to fold to form two vaults, may be dependent on some sort of "material constant." These mechanical properties may be caused by specific biochemical effects within the epithelium that are generated by the metabolism of the cells under genetic control.

From the early bell stages of this study, unfortunately, judgment concerning the just-mentioned hypothesis cannot be made, because these primordia are not sufficiently developed. The occlusal pattern, typical for every single tooth, has not yet formed in every primordium. Therefore, interdependencies between the sizes of the primordia and the number and pattern of epithelial foldings therein cannot yet be evaluated. It may be remembered, however, that for some of the primordia, particularly for i_1 and m_1, there could be found distinctly different outlines of the folded inner enamel epithelium: the casting mold, the *Gussform*, as Ahrens (1913 a) called the primordium in this stage, almost looks like the completed tooth.

Further growth of the dental primordia leads to an increased number of foldings of the inner enamel

12. Here I use the example of molars and premolars, both secondary teeth, because the differences are more graphic; however, the embryological principle may be true for primary teeth as well.

epithelium. As the distribution of mitoses shows (Lefkowitz et al 1953, Paynter et al 1961, Butler and Ramadan 1962, Ramadan-Sadek 1962), the cellular increment is different from region to region and changes in different developmental periods (Ten Cate 1961). In contrast, Glasstone (1939) found no regional differences in mitotic distribution. Development of gestalt of the tooth bell was explained in terms of cellular changes in the enamel pulp (stellate reticulum) (Reichenbach 1928) or in terms of shifting metabolic media in the "diathelial field" (Blechschmidt 1955) of the inner enamel epithelium. Further knowledge has been gained from modern transplantation and explantation experiments (Koch 1967, Kollar and Baird 1969, 1970, Fisher 1971, Lumsden and Buchanan 1986). The main findings from these studies lead to the conclusion that the form of the mesenchymal papilla influences the shape of the epithelium of the tooth bell.

4.5.3 Topography of tooth bells and surrounding bone

One main question of this study is whether surrounding structures (bony structures of the maxilla and mandible, or Meckel's cartilage) may exercise influence in the morphogenetic processes of the tooth germs. From the topographic arrangements in the early bud stage, a spatial impediment as a mechanical factor could be deduced. In contrast, from the topographic relations in the late cap stage, no more mechanical influence seems to be possible from bony structures, because of the relative distance. The same seems to be true for the bell stage, where the overall distance between the primordia and the surrounding hard structures has increased again. The dental primordia thus seem to develop rather independently from mechanical forces from the surrounding structures as soon as they reach the cap stage. The topography of the regionally condensed mesenchyme cannot be discussed here from this point of view, because it was not included in the reconstructions.

Apart from the topography just discussed, an increment of bone in the region between the primordia m^1 and m^2 can be found in the bell stage. There are several other interdental regions, too, in which bony structures increased. In addition, the lingual wall of the mandibular bony groove became thicker in the 64-mm fetus. These are the first signs of formation of the later interdental and peridental bone. Thus, the initiation of bony compartmentation can be found as early as in the 64-mm fetus. Norberg's (1933) study concerned the formation of dental alveolae only in older fetuses of 110 mm CRL and more. In these fetuses, the bony compartments are in a much more advanced stage and may already be called sockets.

5 Final remarks

5.1 Form of the primordia

5.1.1 Early characteristic differences

One of the questions asked in this study was whether the tooth bells, which show some characteristic features of completed incisors, canines, and molars, arise from early buds of more identical "undifferentiated" forms, and attain their characteristic forms to give shape to the different teeth only in later stages of development, or whether, as early as in the bud stage, characteristic differences could be found. The latter case turned out to be true, as the reconstructions of this study reveal. Regional comparison within the same dental lamina arch made it obvious that the single-tooth primordia show specific characteristics beginning from the bud and the early cap stage. It could be expected that the different locations of the dental lamina from which the tooth buds arise may be characterized by specific forms of epithelial swellings. This question, however, requires further reconstructions of earlier laminar stages.

5.1.2 Longitudinal comparison

For the stages from bud to early bell, a longitudinal comparative description can be given for every single tooth.

The primordium of i^1 is round in the early bud stage of the 21-mm embryo, and it retains this form up to the later bud stage in the 37-mm fetus. In the early cap stage, which is reached in the 47-mm fetus, the primordium has become markedly flat in a mesiodistal direction, so that it resembles the later outline of the incisor, the form of which is then retained over the later stages examined in this study. From the reconstructions, no hint can be derived concerning how this alteration of form is accomplished, and no intermediate stage was collected that would have permitted one to follow the transition from the round to the flat form. So far no study can reject the speculation that the overall transverse development of the face in this region may be a reason for the mesiodistal stretching of the incisor primordium.

As for the primordium of i^1 just described, the primordium of i^2 is round in the early bud stage of the 21-mm embryo. In the late bud stage of the 37-mm fetus it is slightly smaller, but still rounder than i^1. In the early cap stage of the 47-mm fetus i^2 has become more oval, but its development with respect to stage and form, lags behind the primordium of the central incisor. The same is true in the later stage of the 64-mm fetus.

The canine primordium c^1 is round in the early bud stage (21-mm embryo), and in the early cap stage, which is reached in the 37-mm fetus, it has attained a triangular outline that becomes more and more distinct with subsequent development.

In the 21-mm embryo the molar primordia are only visible as meager protrusions, which do not permit a reliable description of form. In the 37-mm fetus m^1 tends to be angular, and in the 47-mm fetus it attains a well-defined rectangular outline resembling the later molar shape.

In the bud stage of the 37-mm fetus the primordium of m^2 has an angular outline, which becomes trapezoid by the late cap stage seen in the 64-mm fetus.

In the early bud stage the primordium of i_1 is already clearly flat in mesiodistal direction, as is revealed the reconstruction of the 21-mm embryo. The close proximity of the anterior end of Meckel's cartilage is evident and may be made responsible for the flatness of these primordia. During subsequent stages, the flatness of the primordia of the central incisors is well preserved. However, for the lateral mandibular incisors and those of the maxillary region, it must be assumed that other factors lead to their flattening.

The primordium of i_2 is more rounded in the early bud stage of the 21-mm embryo, and the anterior end of Meckel's cartilage does not expand as far laterally to reach the region of the primordial second incisor. In the early cap stage (37-mm fetus), it has become more oval, although it never becomes as flat as the primordium of the central incisor. In the later stages of the 47-mm fetus and in the 64-mm fetus, it can easily be distinguished from the primordium of the central incisor because of its lesser degree of flatness.

The outline of the canine primordium is round in the early bud stage (21-mm embryo), and, in contrast to the more triangular maxillary canine primordium, it remains rather round in the cap stage in the 37-mm fetus. It becomes triangular in the mature cap stage in the 47-mm fetus, but it is round again in the early bell stage of the 64-mm fetus.

The early bud of m_1 in the 21-mm embryo has an oval shape, which is attained in the cap stage of the 37-mm fetus. In the mature cap stage, it has developed a more pentagonal outline, and in the early bell stage (64-mm fetus), it has a rectangular shape. Here, initial invaginations of the inner enamel epithelium are visible, which may be interpreted as the initiation of fissure and cusp formations.

The primordium of m_2, finally, is an oval protrusion in the 21-mm embryo, and in the 37-mm fetus it has become a bud at the distal end of the dental lamina. In the cap stage of the 47-mm fetus it has a rhombic outline, and in the 64-mm fetus, it has developed an oval, early bell, with its greater diameter in a mesiodistal direction.

5.2 Topography of dental primordia and their surrounding bone

Another task of this study was to elucidate the spatial relationship between the dental epithelium and neighboring structures (in particular, maxillary and mandibular bone, and Meckel's cartilage). As early as the laminar stage, there is a close proximity between some extensions of bony structures and the invaginated oral epithelium. For the transition from the laminar stage to the bud stage, it could be deduced that spatial impediments were one of the factors contributing to the swelling of the tooth buds. The arrangement of Meckel's cartilage and mandibular bone seems to restrict further expansion of the mandibular as well as of the maxillary dental lamina in a dorsal direction.

During further development the distance between bony and dental primordial structures increases (cf Table 3). This may be due to the changes of facial dimensions and proportions that take place during this stage of development. For developmental stages later than the dental cap stage, bony structures should no longer be considered a limiting factor for further extension of the primordia. As far as size is concerned, it could be concluded that there is no interdependency between proximity of bone and size of primordium: primordia that are closer to bony structures (in the anterior region) are generally not smaller than those that have more space in posterior regions, where the bony structures are further away. This posterior region of the primordial dental arch is characterized by a wide distance between primordia and bone, but the primordia of the second molars are the smallest in the maxillary as well as in the mandibular region. In the oldest fetus of this study (64-mm CRL), the primordia of the second primary molars are still much smaller than the primordia of the first, whereas the second molars are the largest in the later primary dentition. It may be true that for the further development of the second molar primordia there is sufficient space for further increases in size. In this context, the introductory assumption of Aristotle, according to which the posterior teeth are larger because they are given more space to expand, is taken up again. The reconstructions of this study, reaching only up to the early bell stage, do not offer a complete solution to this question, but at least it was found that in the 64-mm fetus there is no bone to limit the expansion of the second molars.

5.3 Morphogenesis of the dental primordia

This study did reveal specific patterns of form that in several primordia in stages as early as the bud stage resemble features of the form of the completed tooth. Independently from an increase in size, specific patterns of form such as flatness of incisors, roundness of canines, and rectangularity of molars are retained by some primordia passing through the developmental stages. And as discussed in 5.2, the proximity between the primordia and their surrounding structures cannot be held to be responsible for a morphogenetic influence in the sense of exerting forces to shape the primordia. Possible causes for development of the different forms of the tooth bells should therefore be expected to be found in the primordia themselves. Consequently, on account of genetic factors that are controlling metabolic processes for the expression of form, *the form itself* may be a morphogenetic reason for further development. An overall and equal growth is found only in very few cases. Differential growth, location, and extent of epithelial proliferation or invagination may be dependent on respective initial conditions always found in earlier stages of the primordium. When this principle of gestalt formation is subsequently pursued, it must be assumed that essential information is stored to a certain extent in the earlier stages, even back to the dental lamina stage. Further research is underway to compare exactly the forms of the early swellings of the dental lamina, and to elucidate the spatial relationships leading to formation of the dental lamina.

5.4 Methodological compromise

In this study a detailed investigation of the minute developmental proliferations and movements of tissue during formation of the dental primordia is not possible because the number of reconstructions is not sufficient: intermediate stages, which might be important, could not be collected. Therefore, more reconstructions are required to fill in the gaps in the sequence of developmental stages. In addition, interindividual variations would have to be considered, such as retardation or acceleration of growth and individual deviations of the usual developmental process.

Despite the endeavor to cover the whole developmental process by as many reconstructions as possible, it is impossible to gain a truely *continuous* documentation of development that might lead to generalizations about the developmental process. Our reconstructions are always made from single states of terminated development in different individuals, and to compare their developmental stages is an unavoidable methodological compromise.

In addition, dental primordia reach different developmental stages within the same dental arch, so within an individual, a primordium in the cap stage should not be compared with the adjacent primordium showing a earlier bud stage. Rather, it is necessary to compare the cap stage of one primordium with a cap stage of the adjacent primordium in that of an older individual. However, because of the deficiencies in the collected material, this possibility is not very frequent. We have to be aware of the fact that our reconstructions only show fortuitous "action shots" of an actually continuous process. The present study does supply many new reconstructions and findings, but as a contribution to a presentation of the continuous development of the dental primordia, it is only a humble beginning, despite more than 100 years of research in this field.

6 Summary

It was the aim of the present study to describe the morphogenesis of the dental primordia, covering the stages from lamina to early bell. Regional comparisons between the single primordia along the dental arch were undertaken to work out differences of their gestalt. In addition, the topography and the positional development of the dental primordia in relation of their neighboring structures (maxilla, mandible, and Meckel's cartilage) was described.

For this purpose 18 human embryos and fetuses of a size from 17-mm to 64-mm CRL were prepared as paraffin serial sections. From all specimens serial sections and computer-aided three-dimensional reconstructions were made showing the primordia of the primary dentition and their topographic relations to their surrounding structures.

The following findings can be summarized.

1. In the anterior region, the vestibular lamina and the dental lamina arise from a common epithelial invagination, whereas in the posterior region both laminae are separate invaginations of the oral epithelium.
2. The invaginational depth of the dental lamina varies along the arch and it bears bulgings of different depth and size.
3. Additional and secondary epithelial invaginations of the vestibular lamina were found in the anterior central region in two cases. These additional foldings are not indicative of a so-called prelacteal dentition.
4. Most of the single primordia have a characteristic form from the bud stage onward that possesses features of the completed teeth. Thus, the incisor primordia tend to be flat, canine primordia round or triangular, and molar primordia rectangular or pentagonal. This observation contrasts with the common opinion that the development of form of the specific teeth would not be discernable before the bell stage.
5. The spatial relationship between the dental primordia and surrounding structures like maxilla, mandible, and Meckel's cartilage is different from region to region.
6. From the bud stage onward, all primordia except m^2 are surrounded by a bony groove. The proximity between primordial epithelium and bony structures is as close as 60 μm in early stages, and during further development this distance increases. In the posterior region this distance is usually greater than in the anterior region. The formation of interdental compartmenting bone cannot be observed before the early bell stage.
7. The anterior end of Meckel's cartilage comes very close to the central incisor primordia in the bud stage, whereas it is located below the primordia in the early cap stage.

From the reconstruction of the topographic relationships the following conclusions were drawn.

1. The expansion of the dental lamina is confined in the anterior region by the borders of the face. In posterior direction the mandible and Meckel's cartilage ascend and limit further distal expansion in the mandibular as well as in the maxillary dental lamina. Given further growth, this spatial confinement may be a cofactor in the formation of the tooth buds.
2. Because the distance to the surrounding bony structures increases during development, a morphogenetic influence in the sense of direct mechanical forces may be excluded. However, forces mediated by geometric changes of more remote regions, such as an overall transverse expansion of the face, are discussed as a cofactor of dental morphogenesis.

3. It was found that from the bud stage onward, characteristic features of the outlines are present for several different primordia. It is likely that further development of subsequent stages is dependent on the initial conditions offered by the forms of earlier stages. Thus, the cause of different characteristic tooth forms may be sought in the forms of the earlier buds, if not in the early protrusions of the dental lamina.
4. The present investigation is focused on the morphological aspect of dental development. Although some findings may lead to the conclusion that mechanical factors may contribute to the development of the gestalt of the dental primordia, I am well aware that this is only one part of the mosaic, which, however, should not be neglected. More contributions to factors active in dental morphogenesis are expected from laboratory experimental research that goes beyond the pure morphological description.

Acknowledgments

I wish to thank Professor D. Kubein-Meesenburg, Department of Orthodontics, University of Göttingen, who provided the conditions for me to carry out this study. I am especially grateful to Professor G. Steding and Dr. W. Seidl, Department of Embryology, University of Göttingen, who gave me an understanding of embryology, provided the specimens, and gave very helpful suggestions and ongoing support during the course of the research. For most valuable discussions I thank my friend and coworker, Dr. Andreas Jäger, Department of Orthodontics, University of Göttingen. I also wish to thank C. Mascher, K. von Roden, and H. Sydow for their technical assistance in processing the embryological material.

Following presentation of this study as my habilitation thesis at the University of Göttingen, I thank Professor J. Fanghänel, Department of Anatomy, University of Greifswald, and Professor R. R. Miethke, Department of Orthodontics, Free University of Berlin, for their reports, and Professor G. Steding for his additional votum.

I wish to thank Professor E. Kollar, Department of Oral Biology, University of Connecticut, who encouraged me to publish this study in English after reading the drafts. I am particularly indebted to Dr. B. Freeman, Department of Anatomy, University of New South Wales, for his valuable suggestions in the manuscript stage. Furthermore I wish to thank Quintessence Publishing Co, for their careful reproduction of my drawings.

Finally, I thank my wife, Katharina, and my children, Philip, Kalinka, and Jana, for their forbearance during the years that I spent with the preparation of this work.

This study was supported by grants from the DFG (Deutsche Forschungsgemeinschaft) Ra 428/1–1, 1–2, 1–3, and from the DGZMK (Deutsche Gesellschaft für Zahn-, Mund- und Kieferheilkunde).

7 References

Adloff P. Überreste einer prälactealen Zahnleiste beim Menschen.
Dtsch Mschr Zahnheilk 1909; **27**: 828–832.

Adloff P. Zur Entwicklungsgeschichte des menschlichen Zahnsystems nebst Bemerkungen zur Frage nach der prälactealen Dentition, der sogenannten Konkrescenztheorie und der Entstehung des Säugetiergebisses überhaupt.
Arch Mikr Anat 1913; **82**: 1–37.

Adloff P. Zur Frage der prälactealen Anlagen.
Anat Anz 1913; **43**: 236–238.

Adloff P. Zur Entwicklungsgeschichte des Cervidengebisses, ein Beitrag zur Frage der prälactealen Dentition.
Anat Anz 1914; **46**: 359–366.

Ahrens H. Die Entwicklung der menschlichen Zähne.
Anat Hefte 1913a; **48**: 169–266.

Ahrens H. Entgegnung an Adloff.
Anat Anz 1913b; **43**: 524–527.

Altner G. (ed). *Der Darwinismus – Die Geschichte einer Theorie.* Darmstadt, Wissenschaftliche Buchgesellschaft, 1981.

Anthony F. Anatomie de l'appareil venimeux des reptiles, in de Grasse, PP (ed): Traité de Zoologie, vol 14, 1970, pp 549.

Aristotle. Generation of animals, in Barnes J (ed): *The Complete Work of Aristotle. The Revised Oxford Translation.* Princeton, NJ, Princeton University Press, 1981.

Bateson W. Materials for the study of variation, treated with especial regard to discontinuity in the origin of species. London, 1874.

Baume L J. Einfluß der Funktion auf die Topogenese der Zähne.
Fortschr Kieferorthop 1955; **16**: 315–319.

Blechschmidt E. *Mechanische Genwirkungen.* Göttingen, Germany,
Musterschmidt, 1948.

Blechschmidt E. Entwicklung der Zahnkeime beim Menschen.
Acta Anat 1953; **17**: 207–239.

Blechschmidt E. Rekonstruktionsverfahren mit Verwendung von Kunststoffen. Ein Verfahren zur Ermittlung und Rekonstruktion von Entwicklungsbewegungen.
Z Anat Entwickl-Gesch 1954; **118**: 170–174.

Blechschmidt E. Die Entwicklungsbewegungen der Zahnleiste. Funktionelle Faktoren bei der Frühentwicklung des menschlichen Kauapparats.
Roux's Arch Entwickl-mech 1955; **147**: 474–488.

Blechschmidt E. *Die vorgeburtlichen Entwicklungsstadien des Menschen.*
Basel, Karger, 1960.

Blechschmidt E. *Der menschliche Embryo.*
Stuttgart, Schattauer, 1963.

Blechschmidt E. Der Irrtum des biogenetischen Grundgesetzes.
Fortschr Med 1976; **94**: 465–466.

Blechschmidt E. *Anatomie und Ontogenese des Menschen.*
Quelle und Meyer, 1978.

Böcker F W und Becker R. Zahnentwicklung und Kieferwachstum.
Deutsches Zahnärzteblatt 1965; **19**: 454–462.

Bolk L. Über die Phylogenese des Primatengebisses und das Zukunftsgebiß des Menschen.
Z Morphol Anthropol 1911; **13**: 31–56.

Bolk L. *Odontologische Studien I.*
Jena, Germany, Gustav Fischer Verlag, 1913.

Born G. Die Plattenmodellirmethode.
Arch Mikr Anat 1883; **22**: 584–599.

Born G. Noch einmal die Plattenmodellirmethode.
Z Wiss Mikr 1888; **5**: 433–455.

Brace C L. Structural reduction in evolution.
Am Naturalist 1963; **97**: 39–49.

Burdi A R, Garn S M, Miller R. Mesiodistal gradient of mandibular precedence in the developing dentition.
J Dent Res 1970; **49**: 644.

Butler P M, Ramadan A A. Distribution of mitoses in the inner enamel epithelium of molar tooth germs of the mouse.
J Dent Res 1962; **41**: 1261–1262.

Butler P M. Studies of the mammalian dentition. Differentiation of the post-canine dentition.
Proc Zool Soc Lond 1939; **B109**: 1–36.

Butler P M. The ontogeny of the molar pattern.
Biol Rev 1956; **31**: 30–70.

Butler P M. Dental merism and tooth development.
J Dent Res 1967; **46**: 845–850.

Cope E D. The method of creation of organic forms.
Proc Am Philos Soc 1871; **12**: 229–263.

Cope E D. On the tritubercular molar in human dentition.
J Morph Physiol 1889; **2**: 7–27.

Cope E D. Note on the trituberculite type of superior molar and origin of the quadrituberculate.
Am Naturalist 1883; **17**: 407–408.

Dahlberg A A. The changing dentition of man.
J Am Dent Assoc 1945; **32**: 151–160.

Dahlberg A A. Evolutionary background of dental and facial growth.
J Dent Res 1965; **44**: 151–160.

Dankmeijer J. Eine Methode zur Herstellung mikroskopischer Rekonstruktionen unter Verwendung von Negocoll und Hominit.
Anat Anz 1940; **89**: 81.

de Beer G R. *Embryos and Ancestors.* Oxford, England, Clarendon Press, 1951.

Diekwisch T. *Entwicklungsbiologische Untersuchung über extrazelluläre Matrixproteine, Zytoskelettkomponenten und saure Phosphatase in der Rattenmundhöhle.* Dissertation. Marburg, Germany, 1987.

Dryburgh L C. Epigenetics of early tooth development in the mouse.
J Dent Res 1967; **46**: 1264.

Eidmann H. *Entwicklungsgeschichte der Zähne des Menschen.* Berlin, H. Meusser, 1923.

Elze C. *Zeitschr Anat Entwickl.-Gesch.* 1949/50; **144**: 590.

Eternod A C F. Toute les dents humaines sont des bicuspidées modifées.
Anat Anz Erg-H 1911; **25**: 144–156.

Fisher A R. Morphological development in vitro of the whole and halved lower molar tooth germ of the mouse.
Arch Oral Biol 1971; **16**: 1481.

Fitzgerald L R. Mechanisms controlling morphogenesis in developing teeth. *J Dent Res* 1969; **48**: 726–731.

Florian I, Frankenberger Z.
Embryologie. Prag, 1936.

Gantz S J Z. Studies on the fetal development of the human jaws and teeth.
Dental Cosmos 1922; **64**: 132–140.

Garn S M, Burdi A R. Prenatal ordering and postnatal sequence in dental development.
J Dent Res 1971; **50**: 1407–1414.

Garn S M, Lewis A B, Kerewsky R S. Size interrelationships of mesial and distal teeth.
J Dent Res 1965; **44**: 350–354.

Garn S M, Lewis A B, Vicinius J H. Third molar polymorphism and its significance to dental genetics.
J Dent Res 1963; **42**: 1344–1363.

Garn S M, Lewis A L, Kerewsky R. Shape similarities throughout the dentition.
J Dent Res 1967; **46**: 1481.

Garn, S M. Genetics of dental development, in McNamara J A (ed): *The Biology of Occlusal Development.*
Monograph No. 7, Craniofacial Growth Series, Ann Arbor, Michigan 1977.

Gaunt W A, Gaunt P N. *Three Dimensional Reconstruction in Biology.*
London, Pitman Medical Publications, 1978.

Gaunt W A, Miles A E W. Fundamental aspects of tooth morphogenesis, in Miles A E W (ed): *Structural and Chemical Organisation of Teeth.*
London, Academic Press, 1967, vol I.

Gaunt W A. The vascular supply of the dental lamina during early development.
Acta Anat 1959; **37**: 232–252.

Glasstone S. Regulative changes in tooth germs grown on tissue culture.
J Dent Res 1963; **42**: 1364–1368.

Glasstone S. A comparative study of the development in vivo and in vitro of rat and rabbit molars.
Proc R Soc London Ser 1939; B **126**: 315–330.

Goll R. *Der Evolutionismus.* München, C H Beck, 1972.

Goodwin W K, Cohen M H. A phase-shift model for the spatial and temporal organisation of developing systems.
J Theor Biol 1969; **25**: 49.

Gras H, Killmann F. Neurec – A program package for 3-D reconstruction from serial sections using a microcomputer.
Comput Programs Biomed 1983; **17**: 145–156.

Gras H. A "hidden line" algorithm for 3-D reconstructions from serial sections. An extension of the NEUREC program package for a microcomputer.
Comput Programs Biomed 1984; **18**: 217–226.

Gregory W K. A half century of trituberculy. The Cope-Osborn theory of dental evolution.
Proc Am Philos Soc 1934; **73**: 169–317.

Grüneberg H. The relations of endogenous and exogenous factors in bone and teeth development.
J Anat 1937; **71**: 236–245.

Haeckel E. *Anthropogenie.* Leipzig, 1874.

Hamilton W J, Mossman H W. *Hamilton, Boyd and Mossman's Human Embryology*, ed 4.
Cambridge, W. Heffer & Sons Ltd, 1972.

Harzer W. A hypothetical model of genetic control of tooth-crown growth in man.
Arch Oral Biol 1987; **32**: 159–162.

Hay E D: *Cell Biology of Extracellular Matrix.*
New York, Plenum Press, 1981.

His W. *Unsere Körperform.* Leipzig, 1874.

Ho M W, Saunders P T. Beyond neo-Darwinism – An epigenetic approach to evolution.
J Theor Biol 1979; **78**: 573–591.

Ishizeki K, Fujiwara N, Sakakura Y, Nawa T. The development of mandibular molar tooth germs isografted in the mouse spleen.
Archs Oral Biol 1987; **32**: 695–704.

Jacob M. *Experimentelle Untersuchungen zur Differenzierung des Ektoderm junger Hühnerkeimscheiben.* Dissertation, Göttingen, Germany, 1970.

Kieser J A. Wave superpositioning and the initiation of tooth morphogenesis: an application of the bandwidth theorem.
Med Hypoth 1984; **14**: 249–252.

Koch W E. In vitro differentiation of tooth rudiments of embryonic mice. I. Transfilter interaction of embryonic incisor tissues.
J Exp Zool 1967; **165**: 155–168.

Kollar E J, Baird G. The influence of the dental papilla in the development of tooth shape in embryonic mouse tooth germs.
J Embryol Exp Morphol 1969; **21**: 131–148.

Kollar E J, Baird G. Tissue interactions in developing mouse tooth germs. The inductive role of the dental papilla.
J Embryol Exp Morphol 1970; **24**: 173–186.

Kollar E J, Lumsden A. Tooth morphogenesis: The role of the innervation during induction and pattern formation.
J Biol Bucc 1978; **7**: 49–60.

Kollar E J. The development of the integument: spatial, temporal and phylogenetic factors.
Am Zool 1972; **12**: 125–135.

Korkhaus G. Der Erbeinfluß im menschlichen Gebiß.
Fortschr Kieferorthop 1940; **4**: 189–210.

Kubein-Meesenburg D, Nägerl H, Klamt B. The biomechanical relation between incisal and condylar guidance in man.
J Biomech 1988; **21**: 997–1099.

Kubein-Meesenburg D, Nägerl H, Meyer G, Bücking W. Individual reconstruction of palatal concavities.
J Prosthet Dent 1988; **60**: 662–672.

Kubein-Meesenburg D, Nägerl H, Meyer et al. Zur okklusalen Morphologie. Vergleich der Konturkurven von Front- und Seitenzähnen.
Dtsch Zahnärztl Z 1986; **41**: 21–28.

Kubein-Meesenburg D. *Die kraniale Grenzfunktion des Stomatognathen Systems des Menschen.*
Munich, Carl Hanser, 1985.

Kükenthal W. Über den Ursprung und die Entwicklung der Säugetierzähne.
Jenaer Z Naturwiss 1892; **26**: 469–489.

Kükenthal W. Zur Entstehung des Gebisses des Dugong, ein Beitrag zu Lösung der Frage nach dem Ursprung der Säugetierzähne.
Anat Anz 1914; **45**: 561–577.

Leche W. Studien über die Entwicklung des Zahnsystems bei den Säugetieren.
Gegenbaurs Morphol Jahrb 1892; **19**: 502–547.

Lefkowitz W, Bodecker C F, Mardfin D F. Odontogenesis of the rat molar: prenatal stage.
J Dent Res 1953; **32**: 749–772.

Lumsden A G S, Buchanan J A G. An experimental study of timing and topography of early tooth development in the mouse embryo with an analysis of the role of innervation.
Arch Oral Biol 1986; **31**: 301–311.

Mayr F. *Animal Species and Evolution. Cambridge, 1963.*

McLoughlin C B. Mesenchymal influences on epithelial differentiation.
Symp Soc Exp Biol 1963; **17**: 359–388.

McMurrich J P. The mouth and its organs, in: Keibel, Mall (eds): *Manual of Human Embryology.*
Philadelphia, J B Lippincott, 1912.

Meyer A. *Logik der Morphologie im Rahmen einer Logik der Gesamten Biologie.*
Berlin, J Springer, 1926.

Meyer W. *Normale Histologie und Entwicklungsgeschichte der Zähne des Menschen*, Aufl 2.
Munich, Carl Hanser Verlag, 1951.

Miller W A. Inductive changes in early tooth development: I. A study of mouse tooth development in the chick chorioallantois.
J Dent Res 1969; **48**: 719–725.

Mjör I A, Pindborg J J. *Histology of the Human Tooth.*
Copenhagen, Munksgaard, 1973.

Moss M L. Phylogeny and comparative anatomy of oral ectodermal-ectomesenchymal inductive interactions.
J Dent Res 1969; **48**: 732–737.

Müller G. Die Erbfixation des Gebisses. Versuch einer molekulargenetischen Deutung.
Fortschr Kieferorthop 1975; **36**: 127–134.

Nery E B, Kraus B S, Croup M. Timing and topography of early human tooth development.
Arch Oral Biol 1970; **15**: 1315–1326.

Nilsson T. Zwei Rekonstruktionen als Beitrag zum Studium der Zahnentwicklung des Menschen.
Anat Anz 1928; **66**: 1–6.

Nomata N. A chronological study on the crown formation of the human deciduous dentition.
Bull Tokyo Med Dent Univ 1964; **11**: 55–76.

Norberg O. *Untersuchungen über das dento-gingivale Epithelleistensystem im intrauterinen Leben des Menschen.*
Stockholm, A-B Fahlcrantz, 1929.

Norberg O. Die Morphogenese der primitiven Zahnalveolen beim Menschen und ihre Bedeutung für die Stellungsanomalien der Zähne.
Z Anat Entwickl-Gesch 1933; **100**: 394–432.

Odhner N. Eine neue graphische Methode zur Rekonstruktion von Schnittserien in schräger Stellung.
Anat Anz 1911; **39**: 273–281.

Ooe T. On the development of position of the tooth germs in the human deciduous front teeth.
Okajimas Folia Anat Jpn 1956; **28**: 317–340.

Ooe T. On the early development of human dental lamina.
Okajimas Folia Anat Jpn 1958; **30**: 187–210.

Ooe T. On the development of position of tooth germs in the human deciduous molar teeth.
Okajimas Folia Anat Jpn 1959; **32**: 97–108.

Ooe T. On the development of position of human deciduous molar germs in the latter half of the fetal life.
Okajimas Folia Anat Jpn 1962; **38**: 51–71.

Ooe T. On the position changes during development of human permanent tooth germs in the fetal life.
Okajimas Folia Anat Jpn 1965; **41**: 1–8.

Ooe T. Three instances of supernumerary tooth germs observed with serial sections of human foetal jaws.
Z Anat Entwickl-Gesch 1971; **135**: 202–209.

Ooe T. *Human looth and Dental Arch Developrnent.*
Tokyo, Ishiyaku, 1981.

Orban B. Entwicklung und Wachstum der Zahnleiste und Zahnkeime.
Z Anat Entwickl-Gesch 1928; **85**: 724–733.

Orban B. *Oral Histology and Embryology.* St Louis, Mosby, 1953.

Osborn H F. The history and homologies of the human molar cusps.
Anat Anz 1892; **7**: 740–762.

Osborn H F. Trituberculy. A review dedicated to the late Professor E. D. Cope.
Am Naturalist 1897; **31**: 993–1016.

Osborn H F. *The Evolution of the Mammalian Molar Tooth to and from the Triangular Type.*
New York, MacMillan, 1907.

Osborne R H. Some genetic problems in interpreting the evolution of the human dentition.
J Dent Res 1967; **46**: 945–948.

Paynter K J, Hunt A M. Mitotic activity in rat molar tooth germs.
J Dent Res 1961; **40**: 652.

Pearson A A. The early innervation of the developing deciduous teeth.
J Anat 1977; **123**: 563–577.

Peter K. *Die Zweckmäßigkeit in der Entwicklungsgeschichte.*
Berlin, Julius Springer, 1920.

Peter K. *Methoden der Rekonstruktion.*
Jena, Germany, Fischer, 1906.

Plackova A. Beitrag zum Studium der Entwicklung der Zahnleiste und der Vorhofleiste beim Menschenembryo.
Dtsch Zahnärztl Z 1963; **39**: 265–272.

Poelmann R E, Verbont A J. 3-D reconstructions in anatomy using a semi-automatic device.
Verh Anat Ges 1985; **79**: 155–156.

Preuss F I. Zur Entwicklungsdynamik der Zahnleiste beim Menschen.
Acta Anat 1953; **18**: 283–295.

Provenza D V, Sisca R F. Electron microscopic study of human dental primordia.
Arch Oral Biol 1971; **16**: 121–133.

Provenza D V. *Oral Histology, Inheritance and Development.*
Philadelphia, Lippincott, 1964.

Radlanski R J, Jäger A, Seidl W, Steding G. Zur Frühentwicklung menschlicher Zahnanlagen unter Einschluß der Umgebung. *Dtsch Zahnärztl Z* 1989; **44**: 127–129.

Radlanski R J, Jäger A, Zimmer B. The origin of tooth number of the human deciduous dentition. A hypothesis. *J Med Hypoth* 1988; **25**: 139–140.

Radlanski R J, Jäger A, Zimmer B. The origin of tooth cusps — A hypothesis. *J Med Hypoth* 1988; **25**: 111–114.

Radlanski R J, Kubein-Messenburg D. Embryologische Untersuchungen zur Entstehung der Zahnform. *Dtsch Zahnärztl Z* 1990; **45**: 58–60.

Radlanski R J, Jäger A. Computer-aided 3-D reconstructions (software: HISTOL) in Human embryology applied to tooth morphogenesis. Advantages and limitations, in Smith P and Tchernov E (Eds): *Evolution, structure and function of teeth*. London, Freund Publ, 1992.

Radlanski R J, Jäger A. Zur Lage und Ausdehnung von Epitheleinsenkungen neben Vestibularleiste und Zahnleiste. *Dtsch Zahnärztl Z* 1991; **46**: 305–308.

Ramadan-Sadek A A. *Some Aspects of the Growth and the Differentiation of the Molar Tooth Germs in the Mouse.* Thesis, London, 1962.

Rawles M E. Tissue interactions on scale and feather development as studied in dermal-epidermal recombinations. *J Embryol Exp Morphol* 1963; **11**: 765–789.

Reichenbach E. Die Umwandlung der Schmelzpulpa und der Schmelzepithelien während der Entwicklung des Zahnes. *Z Anat Entwickl-Gesch* 1928; **85**: 490–540.

Rolshoven E. Rekonstruktion histologischer Objekte auf durchsichtigen Werkstoffen. *Z Wiss Mikrosk* 1937; **54**: 328.

Röse C. Über die Entwicklung der Zähne des Menschen. *Arch Mikr Anat* 1891; **38**: 447–491.

Röse C. Über die Zahnentwicklung der Reptilien. *Dtsch Monatsschr Zahnheilk* 1892; **10**: 127–149.

Röse C. Über die Entstehung und Formveränderungen des menschlichen Molaren. *Anat Anz* 1892; **7**: 392–421.

Röse C. Über die erste Anlage der Zahnleiste beim Menschen. *Anat Anz* 1893; **8**: 29–32.

Röse C. Überreste einer vorzeitigen prälactealen und einer vierten Zahnreihe beim Menschen. *Öst-Ung Vjschr Zahnheilk* 1895; **11**: 45–50.

Schour I. Early tooth development with special reference to relationship between the dental lamina and the lip-furrow band. *J Dent Res* 1929; **9**: 699–717.

Schroeder H E. Orale Strukturbiologie, 3 Aufl. Stuttgart, Germany, Thieme, 1987.

Schulze C. *Anomalien und Mißbildungen der menschlichen Zähne.* Berlin, Quintessenz, 1987.

Schumacher G H, Schmidt H, Börning H, Richter W. *Anatomie und Biochemie der Zähne.* Berlin, VEB Volk und Gesundheit, 1990.

Schwalbe G. Über Theorien der Dentition. *Anat Anz, Erg-Heft* 1894; **9**: 5–45.

Scott J H, Symons N B B. *Introduction to Dental Anatomy,* 7th ed. Edinburgh, Great Britain, Churchill-Livingstone, 1974.

Shaw D M. Form and function in teeth, and a rational unifying principle applied to interpretation. *Int J Orthod Oral Surg* 1924; **10**: 703–718.

Spemann H. *Experimentelle Beiträge zu einer Theorie der Entwicklung.* Berlin, J. Springer, 1936.

Starck D. *Biologisches Zentralblatt.* 1949; **68**: 498.

Starck D. Die idealistische Morphologie und ihre Nachwirkungen. *Med Hist J* 1980; **15**: 44–56.

Starck D. *Vergleichende Anatomie der Wirbeltiere III.* Heidelberg, J. Springer, 1982.

Steding G. Die Ursachen der embryonalen Epithelverdickungen. *Acta Anat* 1967; **64**: 37–67.

Stein M R. Polyisomerism of the human dentition. *J Dent Res* 1934; **14**: 125–137.

Sternberger I A. *Immunocytochemistry.* New York, John Wiley and Sons, 1979.

Ten Cate A R. Recruitment in the internal enamel epithelium as a factor in the growth of the human tooth germ. *Br Dent J* 1961; **110**: 267.

Thesleff I, Hurmerinta K. Tissue interactions in tooth development. *Differentiation* 1981; **18**: 75–88.

Thiebold J J, Karcher-Djurichic V, Ruch J V. On the differentiation of odontogenetic fields in mouse lower mandibular arch. *J Dent Res* 1974; **53**: 736.

Thomee S. Über Glasrekonstruktion. *Z Wiss Mikrosk* 1928; **45**: 356.

Tonge C H. The early development of teeth. *Proc R Soc Med* 1953; **46**: 313–318.

Tonge C H. The establishment of individual odontogenic areas in human embryos. *J Dent Res* 1960; **39**: 658.

Tonge C H. Identification of cell patterns in human tooth differentiation. *J dent Res* 1967; **46**: 876–878.

Tonge C H. The time structure relationship of tooth development in human embryogenesis. *J Dent Res* 1969; **48**: 745–752.

Turner E P. The development of the enamel organ in human deciduous molar toothgerms. *J Dent Res* 1959; **38**: 1230.

Turner E P. Early development of the deciduous molar crown pattern in man. *J Dent Res* 1967; **46**: 862–864.

van Valen L. An analysis of developmental fields. *Dev Biol* 1970; **23**: 456.

Waddington C H. *Principles of Embryology.* London, Allen & Unwin, 1956.

Warwick J W. The dental epithelium and its significance in tooth development. *Proc R Soc Med* 1943; **37**: 1–6.

Widdowson T W. *Special or Dental Anatomy and Physiology and Dental Anatomy.* New York, 1948.

Wuketits F. Das Kausalitätsproblem in der Evolutionslehre. *Med Hist J* 1980; **15**: 392–402.

Würtz G. *Zahnentwicklung: Kenntnisstand im Ablauf der Geschichte.* Gießen, Germany, Ferber, 1985.

Yamamura S. Study on primary genesis of human tooth. *J Jpn Stomatognath Soc* 1962; **11**: 16–18.

8 Index

(the numbers in *italics* indicate figures)

additional dentition 65
Aristotle 11, 76
concrescence, theory of 71
cusp formation 70f., 72
dental lamina 14, 21f., *23*, 65
– outline 65
developmental movements 14, 67
differentiation, theory of 71
Dimertheorie (Bolk) 71
enamel chord 52
enamel niche 14, 68
enamel trough 14, 68
evolution, theory of 12, 71
function 12
genetics 13
Genetisches Grundgesetz (Blechschmidt) 65
gestalt 12, 69f.
graphic reconstruction 19
incisor primordium
– maxillary central *25, 29, 30, 37, 43, 46, 53, 56*
– maxillary lateral *25, 29, 32, 37, 43, 45, 53, 57*
– mandibular central *26, 29, 34, 38, 43, 50, 54, 58*
– mandibular lateral *26, 29, 35, 40, 44, 50, 55, 59*
canine primordium
– maxillary *25, 27, 29, 32f., 38, 46, 53, 57*
– mandibular *26, 29, 36, 41, 44, 50, 55, 59*
inductor 13
inner enamel epithelium
– foldings 69, 72
– contour 70
interprimordial distance 67
invagination of the oral epithelium
– onset of lamina formation 63
– pattern 63f., 79
lateral enamel lamina 16
laterale Schmelzleiste 16
law of biogenetics (Haeckel) 65
law of repetitive addition (Cope) 71
Meckel's cartilage 69, 79
merism 72
mesenchymal papilla 73
metabolic fields (Blechschmidt) 71
molar primordium
– maxillary first *29, 34, 38, 43, 49, 54, 57*
– maxillary second *29, 34, 38, 43, 49, 54, 58*
– mandibular first *29, 36, 41, 44, 51, 55, 59*
– mandibular second *29, 42, 44, 52, 56, 60*
morphogenetic field (Butler) 71
natural selection 11, 12
Nebenleiste 14, 40, *38, 43*, 64
occlusal pattern 69f.
prelacteal lamina 64
purpose (of an organ) 11
Schmelzknoten 14
Schmelzmulde 14, 68
Schmelznische 14, 68
Schmelzstrang 52
size and form 72
spatial impediment 14, 66, 69, 77, 79
spatial relationship 66, 73, 76, 79
teleologic view 65
tooth buds 14, 24f.
tooth primordia
– bell stage, early 45f., 69f.
– bud stage 24f., 65f.
– cap stage 34, 37f., 67f.
– cap stage, early 26f.
– lamina stage 21f., 63f.
trituberculy, theory of (Cope/Osborn) 71
vestibular lamina 14, *23*
– additional invagination *31*, 64, 79
wedge epithelium 24, *27*, 66